REFRACTIVE SURGERY

A COLOR SYNOPSIS

Louis E. Probst, M.D.

Medical Director
TLC The Laser Eye Center
Chicago, Illinois
Madison, Wisconsin
Windsor, Canada

John F. Doane, M.D., F.A.C.S.

Refractive Surgeon
Discover Vision Centers
Kansas City, Missouri

Clinical Faculty
Department of Ophthalmology
Kansas University Medical Center
Kansas City, Kansas

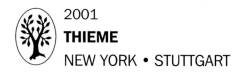
2001
THIEME
NEW YORK • STUTTGART

Thieme New York
333 Seventh Avenue
New York, NY 10001

Consulting Medical Editor: Esther Gumpert
Editorial Assistant: Michelle Schmitt
Director, Production and Manufacturing: Anne Vinnicombe
Marketing Director: Phyllis Gold
Sales Manager: Ross Lumpkin
Chief Financial Officer: Peter van Woerden
President: Brian D. Scanlan
Cover Designer: Kevin Kall
Text Design: Karin Badger
Compositor: Preparé
Printer: Canale

Library of Congress Cataloging-in-Publication Data is available from the publisher.

Important note: Medical knowledge is ever-changing. As new research and clinical experience broaden our knowledge, changes in treatment and drug therapy may be required. The authors and editors of the material herein have consulted sources believed to be reliable in their efforts to provide information that is complete and in accord with the standards accepted at the time of publication. However, in view of the possibility of human error by the authors, editors, or publisher of the work herein, or changes in medical knowledge, neither the authors, editors, publisher, nor any other party who has been involved in the preparation of this work, warrants that the information contained herein is in every respect accurate or complete, and they are not responsible for any errors or omissions or for the results obtained from use of such information. Readers are encouraged to confirm the information contained herein with other sources. For example, readers are advised to check the product information sheet included in the package of each drug they plan to administer to be certain that the information contained in this publication is accurate and that changes have not been made in the recommended dose or in the contraindications for administration. This recommendation is of particular importance in connection with new or infrequently used drugs.

Some of the product names, patents, and registered designs referred to in this book are in fact registered trademarks or proprietary names even though specific reference to this fact is not always made in the text. Therefore, the appearance of a name without designation as proprietary is not to be construed as a representation by the publisher that it is in the public domain.

Printed in Italy
5   4   3   2   1

TNY ISBN 0-86577-914-7
GTV ISBN 3-13-127231-7

To Kate for reminding me that happiness is the real goal.

Louis E. Probst

To Bill and Sara for time lost.
To Sally for all that you have given me and for all that I have taken from you.

John F. Doane

CONTENTS

CONTRIBUTORS

Penny A. Asbell, M.D., F.A.C.S.
Professor of Ophthalmology
Director, Cornea and Refractive Surgery
Mount Sinai School of Medicine
New York University
New York, New York

Kerry K. Assill, M.D.
Medical Director
Sinskey Eye Institute;
National Medical Director
ARIS LASER Vision Centers
Santa Monica, California

Andrea D. Border, O.D.
Optometrist
Discover Vision Centers
Kansas City, Missouri

Dimitrii D. Dementiev, M.D.
Milano, Italy

James A. Denning, B.A., B.S.
Executive Director
Discover Vision Centers
Independence, Missouri

John F. Doane, M.D., F.A.C.S.
Refractive Surgeon
Discover Vision Centers
Kansas City, Missouri;
Clinical Faculty
Department of Ophthalmology
Kansas University Medical Center
Kansas City, Kansas

Lon S. EuDaly, O.D.
Optometrist
Discover Vision Centers
Independence, Missouri

Abdelmonem M. Hamed, M.D.
Lecturer of Ophthalmology

Banha College of Medicine
Sharkia, Egypt

Kenneth J. Hoffer, M.D.
Clinical Professor of Ophthalmology
Jules Stein Eye Institute
University of California Los Angeles;
St. Mary's Eye Center
Santa Monica, California

Debby K. Holmes-Higgin, M.Sc., M.P.H.
Medical Science Communications Specialist
KeraVision, Inc.
Fremont, California

Douglas D. Koch, M.D.
Professor and the Allen, Mosbacher, and Law
Chair in Ophthalmology
Department of Ophthalmology
Baylor College of Medicine
Houston, Texas

Scot Morris, O.D.
Optometrist
Discover Vision Centers
Leawood, Kansas

Mihai Pop, M.D.
Cliniques Michel Pop
Montreal, Canada

Louis E. Probst, M.D.
Medical Director
TLC The Laser Eye Center
Chicago, Illinois
Madison, Wisconsin
Windsor, Canada

Steven L. Ziémba, M.Sc.
Chief Scientist
STAAR Surgical, Inc.
Monrovia, California

PREFACE

Refractive surgery has hit the mainstream. Everyone involved in the ophthalmic industry is being exposed to patients who have had previous procedures or others inquiring whether they are candidates. However, there is a paucity of information that summarizes patient evaluation, the nuances of clinical management, and all the refractive procedures, both past and present, in a readily accessible format. The goal of this book is to fill that void.

Refractive surgery is a visual speciality. Success is measured in the refractive endpoints of uncorrected visual acuity. The preoperative assessment for ocular disease with detailed slit-lamp examination and topography is visual. Finally, the postoperative assessment of the refractive patient requires the correct visual identification of any correctable complications. In order to emphasize the visual nature of refractive surgery, this book has been presented with high-quality representative photographs of essential ocular conditions.

Refractive Surgery: A Color Synopsis is an indispensable resource not only for the ophthalmologist and the optometrist involved with refractive surgery, but also for the ophthalmic technicians, staff, and all members of the eye-care industry who seek a concise yet detailed reference guide that can be accessed in an efficient manner.

ACKNOWLEDGMENTS

We must first thank all the authors for their excellent contributions and assistance with the questions that arose during the editorial process. Without your help, this book would not have come to fruition.

We would also like to acknowledge the tremendous dedication of the Thieme staff, who pulled together to overcome the many obstacles to getting this book done in a timely fashion.

Louis E. Probst and John F. Doane

Options for Refractive Surgery

Louis E. Probst and John F. Doane

CHAPTER CONTENTS

Refractive surgery continues to evolve rapidly with the refinement of procedures and the development of new techniques. The indications for various refractive surgery options continue to change as we uncover the limitations of each procedure through experience and technological advances. A comprehensive approach to refractive surgery requires a clear understanding of the options available to the refractive surgeon.

In 1993, the Casebeer Comprehensive Refractive Surgeon Nomogram summarized available refractive options: radial keratotomy (RK), myopic and hyperopic automated lamellar keratectomy (ALK), photorefractive keratectomy (PRK), and laser in situ keratomileusis (LASIK). Since 1993, the armamentarium of the refractive surgeon has continued to evolve, primarily because of widespread use of the excimer laser for both PRK and LASIK in the United States.

The diagram of options for refractive surgery illustrates the refractive options available to surgeons in 2000 (Fig. 1–1), including laser thermal keratoplasty (LTK), the intracorneal ring (ICR), the phakic intraocular lens (IOL), and clear lens extraction. For the treatment of myopia, LASIK has essentially replaced PRK, which replaced RK as the surgical option of choice. Although myopic and hyperopic ALK have been shown to be effective, myopic and hyperopic LASIK produces more consistent results and fewer technical difficulties. Insertion of the ICR has emerged as an effective procedure for the low range of myopia without astigmatism.

RADIAL KERATOTOMY

Advantages
• effective and relatively economical refractive option for up to 4 degrees of myopia (procedure is adjusted depending on age)

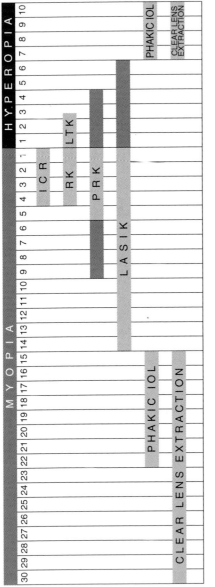

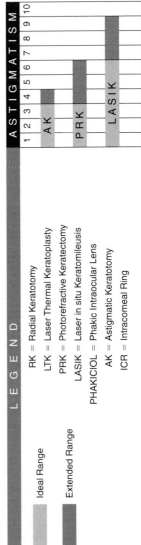

Figure 1–1 This diagram of the options for refractive surgery summarizes the procedures available for the range of refractive errors. As the surgeon gains experience, indications for surgery continue to change. (From: Louis E. Probst.)

Disadvantages
- long-term instability of the refractive error
- reduction of corneal integrity

ASTIGMATIC KERATOTOMY

Advantages
- treats up to 3 degrees of astigmatism
- generally reserved for eyes with a spherical equivalent close to plano

Disadvantages
- often undercorrects astigmatism

AUTOMATED KERATOPLASTY

Myopic Automated Lamellar Keratoplasty
Advantages
- effective for minimal to moderate myopia

Disadvantages
- difficulty making the second "power" cut
- difficult management of the corneal flap
- significant unresolving loss of best corrected visual acuity (BCVA)

Hyperopic Automated Lamellar Keratoplasty
Advantages
- effective for minimal to moderate hyperopia

Disadvantages
- progressive controlled corneal ectasia
- postoperative myopia and irregular astigmatism

PHOTOREFRACTIVE KERATECTOMY

Myopic Photorefractive Keratectomy
Advantages
- more effective for low to moderate myopia and astigmatism

Disadvantages
- corneal haze

- regression
- prolonged postoperative discomfort and need for medication

Hyperopic Photorefractive Keratectomy
Advantages
- treats up to 4 degrees of hyperopia, less than 3 degrees of astigmatism

Disadvantages
- limited to lesser degrees of hyperopia because of possible postoperative regression, corneal haze, and loss of BCVA

LASER IN SITU KERATOMILEUSIS

Myopic Laser In Situ Keratomileusis
Advantages
- effective for low to moderate and (sometimes) high myopia
- rapid visual rehabilitation (1 day)

Disadvantages
- potential flap complications
- regression

Hyperopic Laser In Situ Keratomileusis
Advantages
- effective to at least 6 degrees of hyperopia
- less regression
- little risk for corneal haze
- treats higher degrees of astigmatism (especially when used with an astigmatic scanning excimer laser using cross-cylinder techniques to steepen the flat axis and flatten the steep axis)

HYPEROPIC LASER THERMAL KERATOPLASTY

Advantages
- effective for up to 2.5 D of hyperopia with the Sunrise holmium laser (Freemont, CA)

Disadvantages

- unable to effectively treat astigmatism
- regression (sometimes)
- induces astigmatism ($\leq 20\%$ of cases with retreatment of higher corrections)

PHAKIC INTRAOCULAR LENSES

Advantages

- complete treatment of large spherical refractive errors
- effective for high hyperopia and myopia

Disadvantages

- no treatment of astigmatism
- association of anterior chamber phakic IOLs with endothelial cell loss
- cataracts or anterior subcapsular lens opacities (1–10%, short and long term)
- angle closure and pigmentary glaucoma (rare)
- papillary block glaucoma (rare)
- decentrations (may occur with all phakic IOLs)

CLEAR LENS EXTRACTION

Advantages

- complete treatment of large spherical refractive errors
- effective for treatment of high myopia and hyperopia
- piggy-back IOL insertion allows treatment for extreme hyperopia
- acceptable risk for well-informed patients who are poor candidates for hyperopic LASIK

Disadvantages

- retinal detachment, especially for high myopes (prophylactic treatment of peripheral retinal pathology has reduced risk to the normal lifetime level of 2.4%)

- posterior capsular rupture
- dislocation of the IOL

Suggested Readings

American Academy of Ophthalmology. Automated lamellar keratoplasty, preliminary procedure assessment. *Ophthalmology* 1996;103: 852–861.

American Academy of Ophthalmology. Radial keratotomy for myopia, ophthalmic procedure assessment.*Ophthalmology* 1993;100:1103–1115.

Assetto V, Benedetti S, Pesando P. Collamer intraocular contact lens to correct high myopia. *J Cataract Refract Surg* 1996;22:551–556.

Drews RC. Clear lensectomy and implantation of a low-power posterior lens for the correction of high myopia (discussion). *Ophthalmology* 1997;104:77–78.

Fechner PU, Haigis W, Wichmann W. Posterior chamber myopia lenses in phakic eyes. *J Cataract Refract Surg* 1996;22:178–182.

Koch DD, Kohnen T, McDonnell PJ, et al. Hyperopic correction by noncontact holmium:YAG laser thermal keratoplasty, United States phase IIA clinical study with 1-year follow-up. *Ophthalmology* 1996;103:1525–1536.

Lyle WA, Jin GJC. Clear lens extraction for the correction of high refractive error. *J Cataract Refract Surg* 1994;20:273–276.

Perez-Santonja JJ, Iradier MT, Sanz-Iglesias L, et al. Endothelial changes in phakic eyes with anterior chamber intraocular lenses to correct high myopia. *J Cataract Refract Surg* 1996;22:1017–1022.

Siganos DS, Pallikaris IG, Siganos CS. Clear lensectomy and intraocular lens implantation in normally sighted highly hyperopic eyes: three year follow-up. *Eur J Implant Ref Surg* 1995;7:128–133.

CHAPTER 2

Refractive Disorders

John F. Doane, Scot Morris, Andrea D. Border,
and James A. Denning

CHAPTER CONTENTS

Refractive disorders, also known as refractive errors, are defined as conditions in which the eye does not refract, or bend, incident light to perfectly focus it onto the retina for the best possible visual acuity. The goal of refractive surgery is the elimination of this optical error for excellent unaided visual acuity.

The total refractive power of the eye is the sum of the refractive surfaces of the eye, which include the cornea (the anterior surface, stroma, and posterior surface), crystalline lens surfaces and substance, interface media (e.g., air, the corneal tear film, and intraocular fluid media), and distance separating the individual components of the eye. When the eye optimally focuses incident light onto the foveolar retina, a person has *emmetropia* or no refractive error (Figs. 2–1 and 2–2).

AMETROPIA

Ametropia is the condition in which the eye does not optimally focus incident light onto the foveolar retina. Types of ametropias can be classified by measuring the focusing power of the affected eye or comparing the

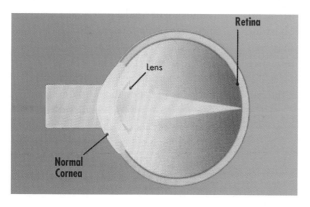

Figure 2–1 Schematic illustrating the condition of emmetropia. The optical elements are set for perfect distance vision without the aid of eyeglasses or contact lenses.

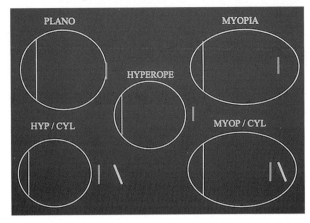

Figure 2–2 Schematics illustrating the five basic refractive states. *Upper left:* In emmetropia, the patient's refractive error is plano. The eye is considered to be spherical, meaning that light bends, or refracts, at all meridians to the same focal plane. In this case, the focal plane is directly on the retina, thus providing excellent unaided vision. *Upper right:* In spherical myopia, either the optical elements (the cornea and crystalline lens) are too refractively powerful or the eyeball is too long, and light is focused in front of the retina (green focal line). *Center:* In spherical hyperopia, either the focusing elements are too weak or the eyeball is too short, and the focal point for the eye is behind the retina (green focal line). *Lower right:* In compound myopic astigmatism, the two major meridians focus in front of the retina and, if regular, are oriented 90 degrees apart. The meridian with the greatest diopter power or ability to bend or refract light (green) is more anterior than the less powerful meridian (yellow). *Lower left:* In compound hyperopic astigmatism, the two major meridians create focal points behind the retina. In this example, the strongest meridian (green) focuses in front of the weaker meridian (yellow).

relative powers of an affected individual's two eyes.

Whether the refractive error of the eye is axial or refractive depends on the length of the eye (axial) relative to normal length or the curvature of the cornea (refractive) relative to average curvature. In *axial ametropia*, the eye is too long or short for its given refractive components. In *refractive ametropia*, the power of the refractive components (cornea and crystalline lens) is too strong or weak for the length of the eye.

Primary Ametropia
- congenital
- hereditary
- environmental
- undetermined

Secondary Ametropia
- trauma (injury of the cornea leading to induced astigmatism or change in curvature, position, or clarity of the cornea or crystalline lens)
- full thickness corneal transplantation (induction of regular or irregular astigmatism, myopia, or hyperopia)
- removal of the crystalline lens (may cause change in corneal curvature at site of surgical wound and result in astigmatism)
- thickening of crystalline lens during aging (leads to more myopic condition)
- clouding or cataract change in crystalline lens (but an intraocular lens may bring the eye close to emmetropia or the desired refraction; small incision surgery results in astigmatically neutral operations)

- scleral buckling procedures for retinal detachment (induction of myopia if the eye is compressed enough to cause axial elongation in anterior-posterior orientation)
- metabolic imbalance (diabetes mellitus leads to a more myopic state and/or fluctuation of refractive error, but condition resolves with physiologic state)

Myopia and Hyperopia

In myopia, or nearsightedness, light focuses in front of the retina (see Fig. 2–2). Conversely, in hyperopia, or farsightedness, light focuses behind the retina (see Fig. 2–2).

Astigmatism

Astigmatism is present when the refractive status of the eye varies depending on which meridian is evaluated. In effect, the focus points for the different meridians do not coincide with each other. Astigmatism may occur with myopia and hyperopia. The total astigmatism diopter power of the eye typically is measured by refraction.

Causes
- corneal astigmatism
- crystalline lens or lenticular astigmatism
- disparity of the line of sight to the optical axis

Astigmatism may be classified according to where one or both major meridians focus light.
- *compound myopic astigmatism*, in which both major meridians focus in front of the retina (see Fig. 2–2)
- *compound hyperopic astigmatism*, in which both major meridians focus behind the retina with accommodation relaxed (see Fig. 2–2)
- *mixed astigmatism*, in which one major meridian focuses in front of the retina (myopic component) and the other major meridian focuses behind the retina (hyperopic component) (Fig. 2–3)

Astigmatism is also classified according to the regularity of astigmatism.

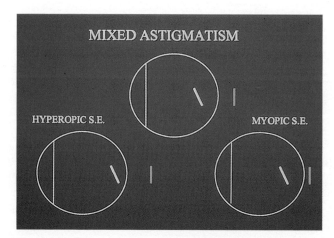

Figure 2–3 Mixed astigmatism. *Upper middle:* The two major meridians have opposite powers, one myopic (yellow) and the other hyperopic (green). *Lower right:* In myopic spherical equivalent (SE) mixed astigmatism, the absolute power of the myopic meridian (yellow) is greater than that of the hyperopic meridian (green). *Lower left:* In hyperopic SE mixed astigmatism, the absolute power of the hyperopic meridian (green) is greater than that of the myopic meridian (yellow).

Regular Astigmatism

- present when the primary (major) strongest and weakest meridians of the eye are 90 degrees apart or at right angles to each other (Fig. 2–4)
- correctable with contact lenses, glasses, or refractive surgery

Irregular Astigmatism

- primary meridians not at right angles to each other and/or the cornea–air interface is not smooth or symmetrical
- less amenable to correction with contact lenses or glasses
- best diagnosed by using a hard contact lens, the rings of a photokeratoscope, or the mires of a manual keratometer to ascertain distortion or irregularity (If a patient sees better with a hard contact lens than with eyeglasses, suspect irregular astigmatism. Rule out defects or opacities as a cause of lost best corrected visual acuity.)

- may be "regular irregular" (prime meridians of curvature that are not 90 degrees apart, sometimes called nonorthogonal, or meridians that are asymmetrical in power across the visual axis) or "irregular irregular" (nonmeasurable fluctuations to the surface that cannot be compensated by a lens)

Presbyopia

Presbyopia is a condition in which the crystalline lens of the eye loses its elasticity and cannot accommodate (change shape) to facilitate near-vision tasks.

- occurs in all patients as they age, typically becoming noticeable after age 40
- reduces the range of clear vision so that no one prescription lens provides clear vision at all distances simultaneously
- eventually leads to the need for bifocal eyeglasses

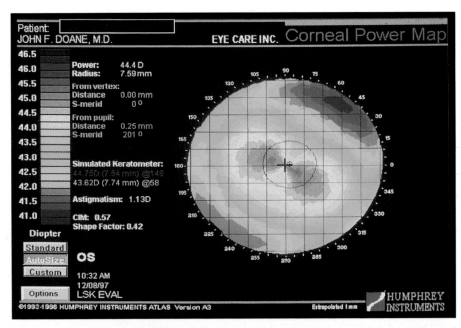

Figure 2–4 Regular astigmatism. The two major meridians are 90 degrees apart from each other and are represented on corneal topography by a typical bow-tie appearance with the long axis oriented along the 148-degree meridian.

REFRACTIVE SURGERY: A COLOR SYNOPSIS

Anisometropia and Antimetropia

Anisometropia is the condition in which the two eyes of a patient have differing refractive powers. With *antimetropia* the two eyes of an individual patient are myopic and hyperopic, respectively.

PATHOLOGIC OCULAR CHANGES AND HIGH REFRACTIVE ERRORS

Patients with significant myopia have an increased incidence of some conditions.
- retinal thinning
- peripheral retinal degeneration
- retinal detachment
- early cataract development

People with extensive hyperopia have an increased incidence of angle-closure glaucoma. Several factors must be considered regarding the incidence of refractive errors. Heredity, the structure of the eye (e.g., myopic eyes have a large axial length and hyperopic eyes have a smaller one), and environmental factors seem to have the strongest influence on the incidence of refractive disorders.

Genetics

Twin and pedigree studies reveal that heredity is a dominant factor in determining refractive errors and disorders.

Environment

Reading and close work have been studied extensively as contributing factors to the induction and/or progression of myopia. Animal experiments have shown an association between onset of myopia and confined living space.

Age and the Structure of the Eye

Longitudinally over time, the refractive error of an individual is not static. There tends to be a natural progression of refractive error as the body changes from infancy through adulthood. Infants and young children tend to be more hyperopic but progress to less hyperopia or frank myopia as they reach adolescence and adulthood because the eye lengthens as it physically matures. Roughly 25% of the adult U.S. population is myopic, but less than 1% of this group has greater than 10 D of myopia. About half of the entire U.S. population over 50 years of age is hyperopic, and of people with myopia or hyperopia, roughly 30 to 40% have concomitant astigmatism.

Ethnicity

Several ethnic groups (Chinese, Japanese, Egyptians, Germans, Eastern European Jews, and Middle Eastern peoples) tend to have a significantly higher prevalence of myopia.

Gender

Subtle differences between the sexes have been reported.
- a slightly higher overall prevalence of myopia in males
- a higher prevalence of myopia that is over −6.00 D in females
- no difference between the sexes as infants
- less difference in children at age 12 than in adults
- refractive changes associated with ocular maturation 2 to 3 years earlier in girls than in boys.

CLINICAL INTERVENTION

The clinician has three options for improving the visual function of a patient with ametropia.
- eyeglasses
- hard or soft contact lenses
- surgery

Suggested Readings

Borish IM. *Clinical Refraction*. 3rd ed. Chicago: The Professional Press, Inc; 1981.

Grosvenor T, Flom MC. *Refractive Anomalies: Research and Clinical Applications*. Stoneham, MA: Butterworth-Heinemann; 1991.

Refractive Errors: Preferred Practice Patterns. 1997; San Francisco: The American Academy of Ophthalmology.

CHAPTER 3

Medical and Corneal Disorders Relevant to Refractive Surgery

Scot Morris, John F. Doane, Andrea D. Border, and James A. Denning

CHAPTER CONTENTS

As we evaluate a patient for possible surgical vision correction, we must consider a variety of conditions, both systemic and ocular, that may affect surgical risk or outcome. A comprehensive systemic and ocular history is crucial for identifying the aspects of these conditions that determine the risks for intraoperative and postoperative complications of refractive surgical procedures. In this chapter, we discuss various systemic and ocular disorders as they pertain to refractive surgery, both preoperatively and postoperatively

MEDICAL DISORDERS

Vascular Disease

The presence of systemic vascular disease should be ascertained during the preoperative evaluation to determine the level of risk associated with refractive surgery. We discuss hypertension and diabetes mellitus, the most common vascular diseases. Other vascular conditions must be considered on an individual basis, with special attention to potential intraoperative and postoperative complications.

HYPERTENSION   Hypertension in refractive candidates is usually mild, well controlled, and rarely associated with significant ocular disease.

Preoperative Considerations
- retinal findings (warrant further evaluation, consideration, and possibly postponement of refractive surgery)
- focal or generalized constriction of retinal arterioles
- arteriovenous (AV) crossing changes
- cotton-wool spots
- flame-shaped hemorrhages
- macular star of hard exudates (HEs)
- arteriolar tortuosity
- intraretinal edema
- preretinal hemorrhage (Fig. 3–1)

Surgical Considerations
- relative contraindications

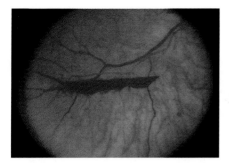

Figure 3–1 Hypertensive preretinal hemorrhage.

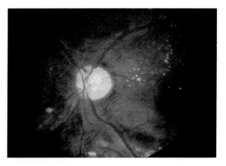

Figure 3–2 Diabetic retinopathy (microaneurysm).

- ◦ lamellar or subconjunctival hemorrhage because of anticoagulant therapy or the presence of corneal pannus
- ◦ effect of hypertension on preoperative or postoperative refractive error or wound-healing processes
- • absolute contraindications
- ◦ sedative cross-reaction with systemic hypertensive medications
- ◦ malignant systemic hypertension

DIABETES MELLITUS Patients with diabetes may be good candidates for refractive procedures if the diabetes is well controlled and the patient's ocular health is good.

Preoperative Considerations
- • systemic history
- ◦ history of blood glucose levels and documented control
- ◦ positive family history of diabetes mellitus
- ◦ presence or history of gestational diabetes
- ◦ history of ocular diabetic findings
- ◦ presence of polydipsia, polyphagia, and polyuria
- ◦ general health status
- • refractive shifts and stability considerations
- ◦ recent unexplained hyperopic or myopic shift

- ◦ refractive instability
- • retinal signs of diabetic retinopathy
- ◦ retinal neovascularization
- ◦ vitreous hemorrhages
- ◦ fibrovascular membranes
- ◦ microaneurysms (Fig. 3–2)
- ◦ retinal hemorrhage (dot blot/hemorrhages)
- ◦ hard exudate
- ◦ cotton-wool spots
- ◦ venous beading (VB)
- ◦ patient education about the progression of diabetes and its possible effect on ocular health and visual function

Surgical Considerations
- • absolute contraindications
- ◦ proliferative diabetic retinopathy (because of the intrinsic risk of retinal disease and loss of visual function with or without refractive surgery)
- • relative contraindications
- ◦ mild to moderate nonproliferative diabetic retinopathy (warrants comprehensive counseling on the potential visual effects of diabetes)
- ◦ increased risk for an allergic reaction to the preoperative sedative
- ◦ anticoagulant therapy
- ◦ moderate risk for lamellar or subconjunctival hemorrhage

Postoperative Considerations
- slower wound healing (because of lower rates of corneal re-epithelialization)
- refractive shifts (require strict blood glucose control and postponement of enhancement procedures until the refractive shifts are stabilized)
- reduced rate of tear secretion and increased risk of dry eye and related symptoms (may require lubricant therapy)

Autoimmune or Collagen Vascular Diseases
This group includes a wide spectrum of diseases with most refractive patients exhibiting minimal signs or symptoms. Preoperative evaluation of the severity of the autoimmune disease as well as the number of medications required is important.

Preoperative Considerations
- decreased tear production because of lymphocytic infiltration and destruction of the lacrimal glands (most collagen diseases)

Surgical Considerations
- absolute contraindications (because of abnormal collagen cross-linking and abnormal and often unpredictable healing processes)
  - scleroderma
  - Marfan's syndrome
  - osteogenesis imperfecta
  - Ehlers-Danlos syndrome
  - documented history of keloid formation [only for procedures like radial keratotomy (RK) and photorefractive keratectomy (PRK), in which there is a prolonged healing process, to prevent permanent haze formation]
- moderate relative contraindications (approach with extreme caution and only after complete patient education about the potential risks of surgery and the long-term visual outcome)

- rheumatoid arthritis
- systemic lupus erythematosus (SLE)
- Wegner's granulomatosis
- polyarteritis nodosa
- relapsing polychondritis
- low relative contraindications (recommend surgery only after complete patient education about possible effects on the healing process and the long-term visual outcome)
  - multiple sclerosis (warrants discussion on long-term prognosis for visual function)
  - conditions that cause iridocyclitis, including ankylosing spondylitis, Reiter's syndrome, and Crohn's or ulcerative colitis (control the condition or wait for latency prior to surgical intervention)

Postoperative Considerations
- increased risk for poor or abnormal healing processes of the ocular surface

Infectious Diseases
Infectious diseases should be treated or stable prior to proceeding with an elective refractive procedure.

HUMAN IMMUNODEFICIENCY VIRUS AND AQUIRED IMMUNODEFICIENCY SYNDROME Many human immunodeficiency virus (HIV)-positive patients are quite healthy and have normal ocular status so they may still be good candidates for refractive surgery.

Preoperative Considerations
- a positive history of HIV or AIDS (does not preclude refractive surgery)
- a thorough history and comprehensive ocular examination to rule out retinopathy
- any sign of acute retinal necrosis, cytomegalovirus (CMV) retinitis, or other HIV retinopathy (warrants discussion about disease progression and effects on vision [Fig. 3–3])

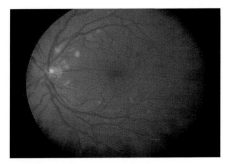

Figure 3-3 HIV retinopathy.

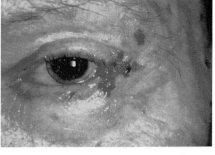

Figure 3-4 Periocular herpes simplex infection.

Surgical Considerations
- need for universal precautions (the Centers for Disease Control provides guidelines) (although no documented cases of transmission of HIV from the tear film or through airborne vaporized particles from laser ablation)

Postoperative Considerations
- need for prophylaxis against postoperative bacterial or herpetic viral infection [fluoroquinolone, as well as trifluridine (Viroptic, Allergan, Irvine CA)], depending on the patient's immune status.

HERPES SIMPLEX Herpetic keratitis often recurs, and residual corneal scarring affects visual performance so careful evaluation and education of these patients are essential.

Preoperative Considerations
- a complete ocular examination and history regarding previous ocular infection
- patient education about proper postoperative hygiene (to reduce risk of ocular contamination and infection for patients with a positive systemic history)

Surgical Considerations
- active ocular and periocular involvement (an *absolute contraindication* [Fig. 3-4])

- previous ocular or periocular infection (a *relative contraindication*)

HERPES ZOSTER AND VARICELLA ZOSTER
Herpes zoster and varicella zoster recur less often but may be confused with herpes simplex infections so precautions are still required.

Preoperative Considerations
- see Herpes Simplex

Surgical Considerations
- latent systemic zoster infection (a *relative contraindication;* advisable to delay surgical correction until the systemic disease is controlled)
  - possible initiation of prophylactic systemic antiviral therapy 1 week before surgical intervention
  - need for universal precautions to prevent contamination (although no documented cases of transmission of virus during laser ablation)
  - increased risk for reactivation and transmission of the viral disease by incisional procedures

BACTERIAL INFECTIONS
Preoperative Considerations
- active infection (treat or control prior to surgery)

Surgical Considerations
- possible postponement of elective surgical correction until signs of systemic disease abate and refractive stability and patient comfort return to normal
- high risk for sedative cross-reaction with systemic antibiotics

Postoperative Considerations
- systemic infection effects on refractive error
- rare medication effects on the refractive error (many medications may cause changes in accommodation)
- effect of sinusitis on patient comfort and tear film (decongestants often decrease normal tear production)

Endocrine and Metabolic Disorders
Few endocrine disorders have a dramatic effect on the eyes and refractive error. Abnormal thyroid function and the intricate hormonal changes associated with pregnancy and lactation are the most common endocrine conditions that may have a notable effect on refractive error and the postoperative healing process. These conditions are discussed in this section.

THYROID EYE DISEASE Patients with mild thyroid eye disease but without significant ocular complications may still be reasonable candidates for refractive surgery.

Preoperative Considerations
- signs or symptoms of thyroid eye disease (displayed by hyperthyroid, hypothyroid, or euthyroid patients)
  - exophthalmos
  - lid lag
  - exposure keratitis
  - diplopia
- binocular status (if binocular abnormalities are noted, educate the patient about possible progression and the potential need for prismatic correction to maintain single binocular vision)
- tear film status (increased likelihood of decreased aqueous secretion secondary to lymphocytic infiltration and destruction of the lacrimal gland)

Surgical Considerations
- refractive instability (an *absolute contraindication*)

Postoperative Considerations
- diplopia (may require prismatic correction after surgery to decrease or eliminate diplopia) (Fig. 3–5)
- tear film stability (may require topical lubricants and/or punctal plugs)

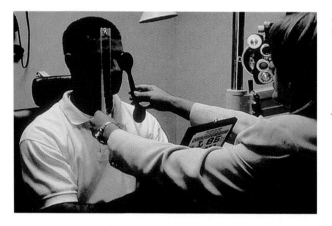

Figure 3–5 Prismatic correction for diplopia.

- dry eye (may require frequent lubrication to maintain comfort and visual function)

PREGNANCY AND LACTATION Patients' refractive stability is often unpredictable during pregnancy and lactation.

Surgical Considerations
- temporary postponement of surgical correction (until after the pregnancy or, if the mother is breast feeding, until three months after weaning)
- potential systemic adverse effects of sedatives and topical prophylactic therapies on the fetus

Postoperative Considerations
- abnormal wound healing
- refractive instability
- tear films abnormality

CORNEAL DISORDERS

Epithelial Disorders
The surgeon and clinician should document various disorders of the corneal epithelium before undertaking surgical intervention. Epithelial basement membrane dystrophy (EBMD) or other epithelial defects may lead to poor or prolonged healing and increased risk for epithelial ingrowth or epithelial defects.

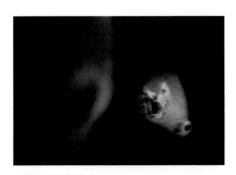

Figure 3–6 Poor epithelial adhesion.

These three processes may lead to patient discomfort during the early postoperative period and increase the risk that further surgery will be necessary. Some surgeons and patients may prefer refractive procedures such as PRK if epithelial disease is present, to prevent postoperative complications and, if possible, treat the ocular surface disease.

EPITHELIAL BASEMENT MEMBRANE DYSTROPHY EBMD is an abnormal maturation and production of epithelial basement membrane with associated abnormal epithelial adhesions.

Preoperative Considerations
- small, cystic, subepithelial, isolated or linear arrangement of subtle opacities (may be observed by focal illumination or highlighted by retroillumination)
- negative staining patterns over abnormal basement membrane

Surgical Considerations
- laser in situ keratomileusis (LASIK)
  ◦ risk for epithelial ingrowth
  ◦ poor epithelial adhesions (Fig. 3–6)
  ◦ difficult flap replacement
- PRK
  ◦ irregular surface ablation
- incisional surgery
  ◦ epithelial ingrowth

Postoperative Considerations
- LASIK
  ◦ epithelial ingrowth formation
  ◦ development of stromal necrosis and flap melt (Fig. 3–7)
  ◦ recurrent erosion because of poor epithelial adhesions
- PRK
  ◦ slow or abnormal re-epithelialization rate
  ◦ recurrent erosions

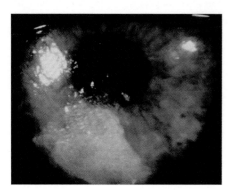

Figure 3–7 Stromal melt after LASIK.

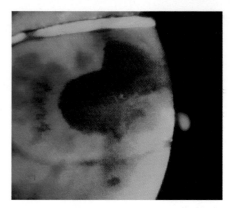

Figure 3–8 Negative staining defect over corneal erosion.

- incisional surgery
  - epithelial ingrowth formation
  - slow or abnormal re-epithelialization rate
- transient changes in vision quality secondary to recurrent epithelial erosions in advanced stages of disease (vision rarely affected in the mild stages of the disease)
- poor lubrication from irregular microvilli formation and subsequent poor glycocalyx formation
- patient discomfort as well as prolonged healing processes (because of the poor attachment of the epithelium small corneal erosions may develop).

RECURRENT CORNEAL EROSION Recurrent corneal erosions (RCEs) are most commonly caused by traumatic injury or other ocular surface disorders that affect the adhesive characteristics of epithelium and its basement membrane to Bowman's membrane.

Preoperative Considerations
- positive history of an RCE (not a contraindication for refractive surgery)
- refractive range
- negative staining defects over recent erosions (Fig. 3–8)
- ocular history of pain upon waking that subsides with time

Surgical Considerations
- poor epithelial adherence in the area of the keratectomy edge or incision
- safety of refractive range (for removal of the area of damaged weak epithelium and basement membrane with PRK)
- preference for PRK or PTK (phototherapeutic keratectomy) over LASIK especially for low myopia with anterior basement membrane dystrophy (allows formation of new epithelial basement membrane and development of normal attachments to the underlying Bowman's membrane or anterior stroma)

Postoperative Considerations
- epithelial ingrowth
- intermittent corneal defects
- poor tear film stability
- patient discomfort

PANNUS OR VASCULARIZATION Corneal hypoxia or inflammation often leads to corneal micropannus or vascularization anterior to the limbus. This vascularization is common in those who overwear their contact lenses or in the presence of other ocular surface diseases.

Preoperative Considerations
- any effect of the pannus on the visual axis

Surgical Considerations

- proximity to incision or keratectomy (Fig. 3–9) (may lead to intralamellar hemorrhage)
- intraoperative hemorrhage
- flap retraction along edge of pannus

Postoperative Considerations

- intralamellar hemorrhage
  - inflammatory reaction (resulting in intralamellar keratitis)
  - localized edema (resulting in decreased vision)
- vascular advancement into the incisions
- hemosiderin deposition
  - decreased vision from localized inflammatory process and edema
  - intralamellar keratitis

MEESMAN'S AND REIS BUCKLER CORNEAL DYSTROPHIES Meeseman's or hereditary juvenile epithelial dystrophy is a bilateral and symmetric formation of epithelial cysts with thickened basement membrane that appear as early as the first few months of life. Reis Buckler disorder is a Bowman's membrane disorder that also affects the central cornea. It is a bilateral and symmetric condition that usually results in central corneal opacities and a subsequent decrease in visual function by the first to second decades of life.

Surgical Considerations

- need for a lamellar or full thickness corneal graft in advanced stages to

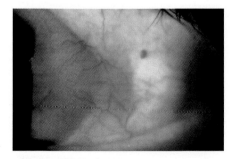

Figure 3–9 Pannus close to an RK incision.

decrease the fibrillar material that has replaced Bowman's membrane (an *absolute contraindication* for lamellar refractive surgery)

Stromal Disorders

Most stromal disorders are relative contraindications for refractive surgery, though patients with some stromal dystrophies may benefit to some degree from lamellar surgery. A few stromal disorders, including ectatic disorders such as keratoconus are absolute contraindications for refractive surgery.

KERATOCONUS The etiology of keratoconus is unknown, but the progressive thinning of the central cornea associated with this disorder presents obvious challenges to successful refractive surgery.

Preoperative Considerations

- topography (for all refractive patients)
- pachymetry (for all patients in whom central corneal thinning is suspected)
- early-stage findings
  - subtle, irregular astigmatism, usually bilateral but asymmetric [central corneal curvature readings of >48 D (Fig. 3–10) and vertical asymmetry >5 D (Fig. 3–11)]
  - progressive myopia (usually bilateral but asymmetric)
  - moderate-stage findings
  - progressive thinning of the central cornea (central corneal thickness significantly lower than peripheral corneal thickness, commonly <500 μm)
  - Fleischer's ring
  - Vogt's stria

Surgical Considerations

- an *absolute contraindication* to all current types of refractive surgery because progressive corneal thinning increases the risk of corneal instability

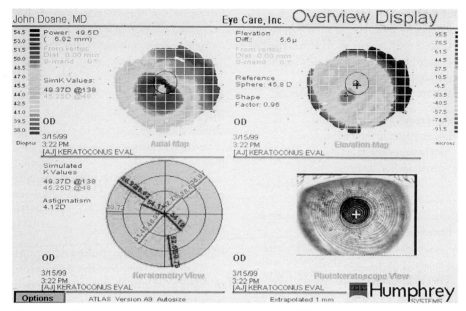

Figure 3–10 Topography with corneal curvature greater than 48 D.

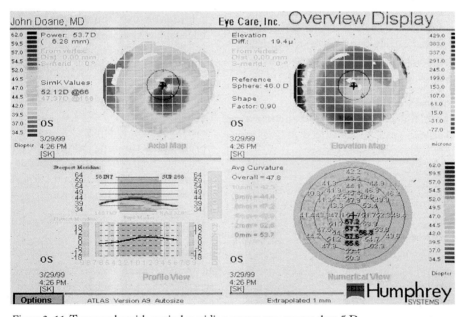

Figure 3–11 Topography with vertical meridian asymmetry greater than 5 D.

THIN CORNEAS Corneal thickness measurements are critically important for determining risk for both incisional and lamellar refractive surgery. The surgeon must both rule out preoperatively and prevent the development postoperatively of corneal ectasia.

Preoperative Considerations
- assessment of corneal thickness by pachymetry (average corneal thickness in normal myopic patients = 545–555 μm)
  - minimization of postoperative risk for iatrogenic keratoconus (from lamellar surgery)
  - minimization of postoperative risk for full-thickness perforations and endophthalmitis (from incisional surgery)
- estimated postoperative stromal bed thickness (for lamellar surgery)
  - ideal = ≥ 300 μm
  - borderline = 250 μm
  - absolute minimum = 200 μm
- variations in lamellar flap thickness (flat corneal curvature may result in an abnormally thin cap)

Surgical Considerations
- incisional surgery
  - number of incisions (affected by corneal thickness)
  - corneal thickness determines depth of incisions (perforations at any location during surgery suggest excessive incisional depth)
- lamellar surgery
  - estimation of postoperative corneal thickness (preoperative corneal thickness— thickness of stromal tissue ablated), which determines ablation profile and multizone vs. single zone considerations
  - thin cap or a perforation in the corneal cap

Postoperative Considerations
- signs of corneal perforation after incisional surgery

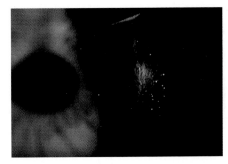

Figure 3–12 Gaping RK incision.

  - positive Seidel's sign
  - gaping incisions (Fig. 3–12)
  - localized deep stromal inflammation and edema
  - endophthalmitis
- lamellar surgery
  - corneal ectasia from an abnormally thin cornea
  - irregular astigmatism
  - progressive myopia
  - postoperative evaluation for iatrogenic keratoconus (thin corneas with refractive instability and steepening on topography, including pachymetry and topography)

STROMAL OPACIFICATION OR SCARS Stromal scars may be insignificant if completely off the visual axis or very significant if within the visual axis. Scars in the visual axis may cause a loss of BCVA and often lead to a suboptimal postoperative result.

Preoperative Considerations
- opacity (evaluated by slit lamp exam)
  - depth
  - location [effect on visual axis (Fig. 3–13)]
  - density
  - effect on refractive error assessment

Surgical Considerations
- selection of appropriate surgical procedure

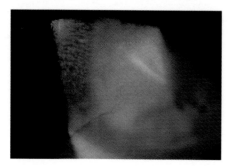

Figure 3–13 Stromal scar near the visual axis.

○ potential effect of the opacity or fibrosis depth on ablation profile
○ probability of removal or decrease in density of opacity or fibrosis with refractive procedure
• incisional surgery
○ for opacities outside the visual axis (opacity will not affect postoperative healing of the incisions)
○ irregular wound healing (effect of fibrosis on radial keratectomy blade incision)
○ difficulty creating channel for insertion (effect of opacity or fibrosis on intracorneal ring insertion)
• lamellar surgery
○ LASIK indicated when the opacity is outside the visual axis (opacity will not affect postoperative healing of the flap)
○ risk for irregular ablation (effect of the opacity or fibrosis on ablation profiles and homogeneity of ablation)
• intraocular surgery (if the opacity is outside the visual axis)
○ difficult visualization of anterior segment

Postoperative Considerations
• wound healing
○ irregular healing and/or increased fibrosis (effect of opacity or fibrosis depth)

○ irregular healing at fibrosis location (effect of opacity or fibrosis location)
○ potential increase in fibrosis density if incision passes through fibrosis (effect of opacity or fibrosis density)
• visual acuity (development of irregular astigmatism or surface changes)
○ irregular healing with potential irregular astigmatism (effect of opacity or fibrosis depth)
○ effect of opacity or fibrosis density (see above)
• partial-thickness lamellar graft (may eliminate the opacity and enhance unaided visual acuity)

STROMAL DYSTROPHIES The three primary stromal dystrophies (lattice, macular, granular) are not contraindications for refractive surgery but may pose difficulty in both presurgical evaluation and surgical performance.

Preoperative Considerations
• evaluation of cornea to identify stromal dystrophy
• effects of stromal dystrophy
• refractive error (more difficulty getting a refractive endpoint)
○ visual acuity (BCVA may be reduced because of stromal opacities)
○ potential for reduced preoperative BCVA
• patient education
○ risks of surgery
○ diagnosis of stromal dystrophy
○ potential effect on visual acuity
○ risk for disease progression and long-term visual acuity

Surgical Considerations
• ablation profile alterations (deeper ablation to remove opacities)
• intraoperative hydration levels (different hydration pattern of stroma because of different components)

- incisional difficulty (because of difficult visualization and different consistency of stroma)

Postoperative Considerations
- delay in healing response
- initial reduction in visual acuity because of poor healing response
- ocular surface abnormalities

Endothelial Disorders

Although less common, endothelial corneal dystrophies comprise a complex group of conditions that may significantly impact the results of refractive surgery. Patients should be carefully screened for these conditions before undergoing any refractive discussion.

ENDOTHELIAL GUTTATA OR FUCHS' DYSTROPHY A few endothelial guttata are commonly found in patients older than 60 years of age and represent a premature aging process involving the corneal endothelium. Fuchs' dystrophy is the association of guttata with frank corneal edema indicating endothelial decompensation (an absolute contraindication to refractive surgery).

Preoperative Considerations
- dewdrop or wartlike endothelium excrescences in the central cornea
  - indicates an overall weakness of the corneal endothelium
  - must be differentiated from endothelial pigment that is often deposited in the same location
  - endothelial cell counts should be considered prior to any refractive procedure [if >10 guttata or if an intraocular procedure, such as phakic intraocular lens (IOL) insertion or clear lens extraction, is being considered]
- presence and status of corneal edema

Surgical Considerations
- good visual acuity and good prognosis for corneal integrity (then *not* a contraindication for refractive surgery)
- presence or severity of guttata

Postoperative Considerations
- visual acuity (edema and excessive corneal hydration may produce a myopic shift)
- corneal edema (minimize with hypertonics)
- damage to ocular surface integrity
  - artificial tears or lubricating ointment
  - bandage hydrogel lens (if necessary)

Other Corneal Disorders

Preoperative identification of other rare corneal dystrophies is important because they may impact surgical planning and results of refractive procedures.

Preoperative Considerations
- examination to exclude posterior polymorphous dystrophy and iridocorneal endothelial dystrophies

Surgical Considerations
- absolute contraindications
  - posterior polymorphous dystrophy
  - iridocorneal endothelial dystrophies
  - infectious keratitis with active herpetic infection or active fungal infection
- relative contraindications
  - active bacterial infection (postpone surgery until the ocular surface is clear)
  - past history of herpetic infection (surgery carries a risk of reactivation; provide prophylactic treatment)

Postoperative Considerations
- continuation of antiviral therapy if past herpetic infection is suspected
- monitoring of intraocular pressure (IOP) every 6 months if iridocorneal dystrophies suspected

DISORDERS OF OTHER OCULAR STRUCTURES

Eyelids

Eyelid abnormalities must be evaluated, documented, and managed properly to ensure the best possible surgical outcome. Ptosis, blepharitis, and appositional or meibomian gland disorders may affect patients' intra- and postoperative status and are discussed in the following sections.

PTOSIS Mild ptosis (eyelid droop <1 mm should be documented whenever noted preoperatively.

Preoperative Considerations
- proper assessment and documentation of preexisting ptosis (useful as a reference if its preexisting status is questioned after surgery)
- history of lid surgery or trauma (may indicate reason for ptosis and document that refractive procedure did not cause it)
- decreased levator function (may be associated with poor lid closure and exposure after refractive procedures)
- narrowing of the palpebral fissure (more difficult access to the eye for procedures)

Surgical Considerations
- proper and careful speculum placement (may cause further damage to the lid muscles, particularly if there was recent lid surgery)

Postoperative Considerations
- temporary ptosis (levator function usually returns within a few days but necessitates education of patient about cause and duration)
- permanent but rare ptosis (may warrant surgical repair for the following reasons)
  ○ cosmetically unacceptable
  ○ incomplete lid closure causing exposure keratitis

○ reduction of visual field or blocking of visual access by lid

BLEPHARITIS Blepharitis is a very common eyelid condition often associated with dry eyes and meibomian gland dysfunction.

Preoperative Considerations
- proper diagnosis of and differentiation between staphylococcal and seborrheic blepharitis
- evaluation of dry eyes
- evaluation of any keratitis secondary to the blepharitis or dry eyes
- bulbar conjunctival edema
- anterior blepharitis
  ○ *Staphylococcus* sp. flakes on the base of the eyelashes (collarettes), eyelid ulceration, associated marginal keratitis (preoperative treatment reduces risk of infection)
- posterior blepharitis
  ○ chalazion (infection of meibomian gland; use lid scrubs and ocular lubrication generously for several weeks to eliminate prior to refractive surgery)
  ○ seborrheic secretions on eyelashes (sleeves) associated with scalp dandruff (Fig. 3–14)

Surgical Considerations
- reduction or elimination of risk for postoperative infectious keratitis by postpon-

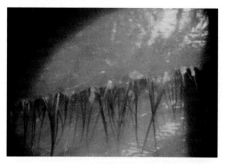

Figure 3–14 Seborrheic blepharitis.

ing any procedure until blepharitis is controlled
- bulbar conjunctival edema and difficult keratome placement
- proper irrigation of the surgical field with topical antibiotics to prevent infection
- minimal contact with affected lids (if possible)

Postoperative Considerations
- incisional surgery
  - endopthalmitis induced by corneal perforation (treat aggressively)
  - corneal ulceration (treat aggressively with fluoroquinolones and monitor daily)
- lamellar surgery
  - intrastromal keratitis caused by bacterial endotoxin (treat with topical antibiotics, steroids, or both; usually clears within a few weeks, even if left untreated)
  - corneal ulceration (treat aggressively with fluoroquinolones)

MEIBOMIAN GLAND DYSFUNCTION Abnormal production, constitution, or secretion of lipid from the meibomian glands characterizes meibomian gland dysfunction (MGD).

Preoperative Considerations
- indentification of chalazion

Surgical Considerations
- presence of chalazion (an *absolute contraindication*)
  - may alter corneal structure and refractive status
  - may affect patient comfort during and after surgery
  - treat appropriately before surgical intervention
- careful speculum placement to avoid excess lipid excretion or patient discomfort

- proper irrigation to eliminate lipid deposits in the lamellar interface in LASIK and PRK

Postoperative Considerations
- ocular surface inflammation
- mild intrastromal keratitis
- patient discomfort

Conjunctival Abnormalities
Preoperative Considerations
- conjunctival chemosis (Fig. 3–15)
- conjunctival redundancy
- conjunctival inflammation

Surgical Considerations
- absolute contraindication
  - infectious conjunctivitis
- relative contraindications
  - conjunctival redundancy or chemosis (proper vacuum for the keratectomy is often difficult in lamellar surgery)
  - generalized conjunctival inflammation (may lead to poor healing response in intraocular surgery)

Postoperative Considerations
- wound healing complications (swollen inflamed conjunctiva may lead to an uneven ocular surface that prevents the smooth flow of tears and medications)
- infectious conjunctivitis (treat aggressively)

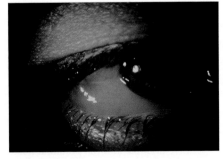

Figure 3–15 Conjunctival chemosis.

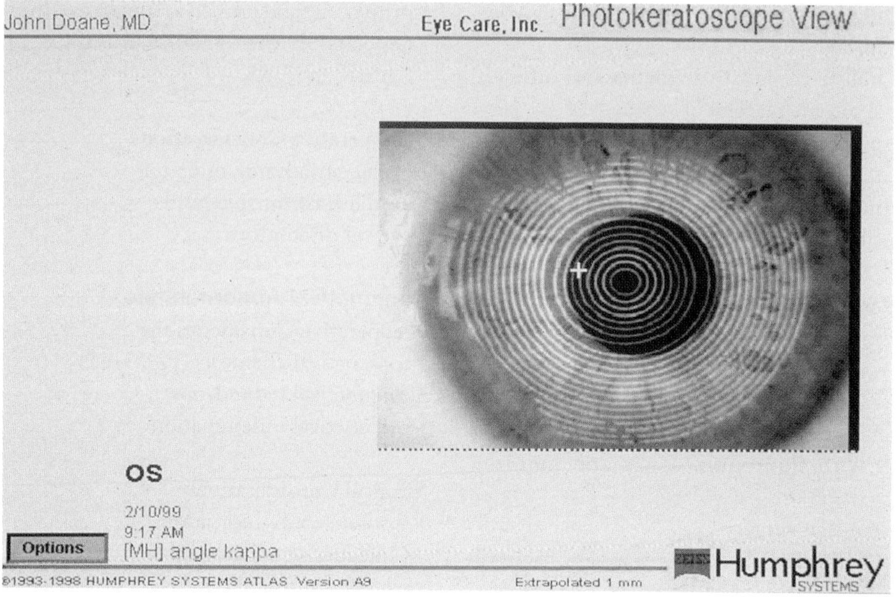
John Doane, MD
Eye Care, Inc.
Photokeratoscope View
OS
2/10/99
9:17 AM
[MH] angle kappa
Options
©1993-1998 HUMPHREY SYSTEMS ATLAS Version A9
Extrapolated 1 mm
Humphrey
SYSTEMS

Figure 3–16 Angle kappa as seen on topography (photokeratoscopic view).

- ocular discomfort
  - resolves in 24 to 48 hours
  - often responds to postoperative steroid drops

Extraocular Muscles

Phorias and tropias present an interesting challenge to the refractive surgeon because they are often corrected with a prism in the patient's glasses. Patients often assume that the refractive procedure can also eliminate this prism, which is not possible. Preoperative counseling and potential treatment of the phoria or tropia is required.

Preoperative Considerations

- identification of motility or binocular status abnormalities for proper alignment of the visual system and successful surgical and visual outcome
- patient education about the risk for postoperative diplopia and the potential need for postoperative prismatic correction
- phorias (rarely affect intraoperative or postoperative outcomes of refractive procedures)
- tropias
  - may affect visual outcome and overall subjective success of the surgery
  - significant surgical correction before the refractive procedure may be indicated
- angle kappa (Fig. 3–16) (usually identified in hyperopic patients via photokeratoscopy and topography [photokeratoscopic view])

Surgical Considerations

- possible poor intraoperative fixation resulting from tropias
- alignment of visual axis (crucial for proper centration and central optical zone determination in incisional surgery)
- lamellar surgery
  - alignment of visual axis
  - patient fixation
  - ablation centration (Fig. 3–17)

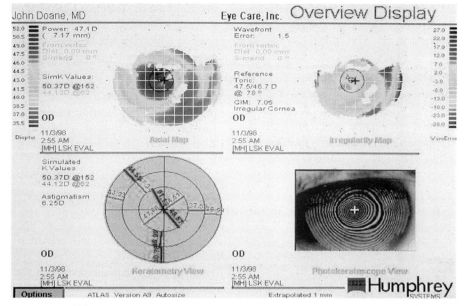

Figure 3–17 Ablation centration in the presence of angle kappa.

Postoperative Considerations
- aggravation of the binocular status of some patients can result in subjective or objective diplopia
- reduction or elimination of certain binocular problems by elimination of the refractive error for some patients
- postoperative diplopia secondary to removal of prismatic or accommodative effect of the spectacle lens with tropia
  - visual therapy (if indicated)
  - prismatic spectacle correction
  - surgical correction of the tropia (misalignment) in rare cases

Large Pupils
Preoperative Considerations
- evaluation of pupil size (using scotopic and photopic illumination, to avoid postoperative complaints about glare)
- choice of ablation zone of the laser (should be at least as big as the scoptic pupil size)
- preoperative perception of glare (thorough history with and without correction)

- patient counseling about the risk of postoperative glare

Surgical Considerations
- proper alignment of the visual axis and the pupil (essential to successful surgical and visual outcome)
- choice of the biggest zone possible

Postoperative Considerations
- "off-axis" treatment of persistent complaints of diplopia or scotopic glare
- spectacle tint or specialized contact lens to decrease glare

Orbital Configuration and Palpebral Opening
In lamellar surgery, small or deep-set eyes may make it difficult for the surgeon to set the microkeratome ring in the proper position. Narrow fissures also may make it difficult to place the ring, or may interfere with microkeratome movement. Unusual orbital configuration/palpebral openings

also may increase postoperative patient discomfort because of lid trauma during surgery.

INCOMPLETE EYELID CLOSURE Patients may have nocturnal lagophthalmos and are often unaware that they have the condition. A careful preoperative examination allows anticipation and postoperative treatment of exposure problems if necessary.

Preoperative Considerations
- inferior band staining greater in the morning
- visible scleral show when eyelids are gently closed

Surgical Considerations
- proper speculum selection (allows for proper positioning with minimal patient discomfort)
- minimal anesthesia
- copious lubrication

Postoperative Considerations
- exposure keratitis (occurs often but is treatable with lubricants)
- use of ocular lubricants
- punctal plugs
- taping of eyelid at night for first week after procedure

SMALL FISSURE SIZE Hyperopic eyes in particular are associated with small fissures. The smaller opening makes any surgical procedure more difficult because visualization is more difficult and the equipment is a standard size.

Preoperative Considerations
- appropriate measurement of fissures to assess preoperative interpalpebral opening size (for LASIK, test the fit of the suction ring in the eye)
- patient education about difficulty of surgery on eyes with small fissures

Surgical Considerations
- proper speculum selection to increase patient comfort
- keratome selection for ease of passage

Postoperative Considerations
- usually minimal postoperative visual effects

Retinal Disorders
Retinal disorders should be evaluated and treated so that they are completely stable for any elective refractive procedure.

Preoperative Considerations
- identification of retinal tears, holes, detachment, or retinal scars
- history of retinal detachment
- history of previous retinal surgery

Surgical Considerations
- absolute contraindication
  ○ visually threatening retinopathy
- relative contraindications (preoperative repair indicated)
  ○ untreated retinal breaks
  ○ retinal holes
  ○ retinal tears
- careful placement of suction ring detachment to ensure adequate suction (if previous scleral buckle for retinal detachment)

Postoperative Considerations
- follow-up for all retinal pathology (greater risk for retinal detachment continues to be present)

Suggested Readings

Doane JF, Slade SG. ALK, LASIK, and hyperopic LASIK. In: Wu H, Steiner R, Slade S, Thompson V, ed. *Refractive Surgery.* New York: Thieme; 1999:393–406.

Machat JJ. Preoperative myopic and hyperopic LASIK evaluation. In: Machat JJ, Slade SD, Probst LE, ed. *The Art of LASIK.* Thorofare, NJ: Slack Inc.; 2000:127–138.

Slade SG, Doane JF, Ruiz LA. Laser myopic keratomileusis. In: Elander R, Rich LF, Robin JB, ed. *Principles and Practice of Refractive Surgery.* Philadelphia: W.B. Saunders; 1997: 357–366.

Thompson VM, Wallin D. Patient selection and preoperative considerations. In: Wu H, Steiner R, Slade S, Thompson V. *Refractive Surgery.* New York: Thieme; 1999:41–52.

CHAPTER 4

Preoperative Assessment

Scot Morris, John F. Doane, Andrea D. Border,
James A. Denning, and Louis E. Probst

CHAPTER CONTENTS

The quality of our vision continually affects every one of us regardless of occupation, age, sex, economic situation, or marital status. Vision dramatically shapes our perceptions, and for many individuals, vision is the primary means of interpreting the world around them. Each individual places a different value on the status and importance of vision. Clinicians and surgeons must remember to carefully and accurately assess not only each individual's medical eligibility but also his or her expectations and demands. Each patient interested in undergoing refractive surgery should have a thorough examination that includes a comprehensive history and ocular exam.

REASONS FOR SEEKING REFRACTIVE SURGERY

Ascertaining each patient's reasons for pursuing refractive surgery is crucial to the ultimate success of the procedure.

Common Patient Characteristics
• young to middle aged
• well educated
• professional
• successful
• type A personality
• potential for loss of income if vision compromised

Occupational Needs and Restrictions

INHERENT RISK OF SPECTACLE WEAR In some employment situations, vision correction with eyeglasses may pose inherent safety or health risks.
• lost, broken, or otherwise damaged eyeglasses (common in civil protection jobs, leaving the individual unable to see or function effectively and potentially placing the person or others in harm's way)
• hindrance of excellent peripheral vision needed for certain jobs (e.g., construction workers, police officers, or firefighters)

• difficulties with bifocals for presbyopic individuals who are confronted with tasks that require multiple fixation distances (e.g., nurses, teachers, or office managers)

INHERENT RISK OF CONTACT LENSES
Some work environments are particularly hazardous to contact lens wearers. For example, firefighters frequently encounter smoke and a police officer could lose his or her contacts during a physical confrontation.
• toxic chemicals infiltrating contact-lens material or affecting the ocular surface
• direct or indirect exposure to biohazards and potential for ocular damage
• desiccation from arid work conditions
• airborne foreign particles that may be trapped under the lens

NEED FOR UNAIDED VISUAL ACUITY
Many professions are restricted to individuals with certain levels of uncorrected visual acuity. Although several of the policies that regulate these professions are now being challenged, individuals must research predicted outcomes, inherent risks, and possible exclusions for employment.
• branches of the military
• commercial airline pilots
• certain civil protection agencies and groups (e.g., Navy SEALs, the FBI, state troopers, local police officers)
• jobs with restrictive environmental or safety conditions
• jobs with policies denying employment to individuals who have previously undergone refractive surgery (generally because of concern about unstable vision and degradation of visual acuity at night)

Recreational Needs
• restriction of athletic activities because of eyeglasses
  ◦ loss of peripheral vision from frames

◦ problems switching from near to far focus with bifocal eyeglasses
• problems with contact lenses
  ◦ desiccation
  ◦ intolerance of chlorine in swimming pools when wearing contact lenses
  ◦ submersion and potential loss of contact lenses during water sports
  ◦ loss of independence if eyeglasses or contact lenses are broken or lost

COSMETIC AND PERSONAL NEEDS
Regardless of what we view as critical, some patients perceive wearing eyeglasses or contact lenses as threatening to their lifestyles and occasionally their lives or health.
• elimination of red or dry eyes from contact lens wear
• elimination of social stigma associated with thick spectacle lenses (Fig. 4–1)
• enhancement of personal appearance
• need for more youthful look during a "mid-life crisis"
• elimination of reading glasses and multiple pairs of readers
• perceived threat to life without adequate visual acuity if eyeglasses or contacts are lost during an emergency
• avoidance of conditions unfavorable for contact lens wear

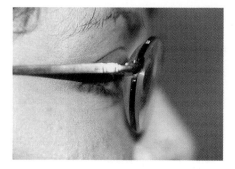

Figure 4–1 Example of thick spectacle lenses that may stigmatize the wearer.

SPECTACLE INTOLERANCE Some patients consider refractive surgery because they have problems wearing eyeglasses.

- uncomfortable spectacle wear because of a narrow bridge (Fig. 4–2) or wide face and improper frame width
- allergic reaction to the frame materials
- lens condensation with temperature changes
- frame slippage because of perspiration on the bridge
- poor vision from improper lens design, lens or bifocal fit, or an incorrect prescription

CONTACT LENS INTOLERANCE Other patients consider refractive surgery to avoid wearing contact lenses.

- dry eyes, which may lead to reduced wearing time, redness, and irritation
- hypersensitivity to lens cleaning and moistening solutions
- poor vision secondary to uncorrected astigmatism because of spherical lenses
- increased dependence on reading glasses by prepresbyopes even with contact lens wear

PRESBYOPIA

- elimination of readers through hyperopic and hyperopic astigmatic laser ablation

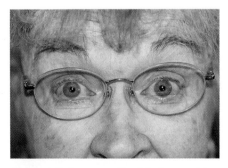

Figure 4–2 An uncomfortable frame with a narrow bridge.

(allows ametropic individuals to undergo monovision correction)

- decreased dependence on reading glasses through monovision applications

REASONS FOR *NOT* SEEKING REFRACTIVE SURGERY

Equally as important as patients' reasons for pursuing refractive surgery are their reasons for avoiding surgery. A successful surgical outcome mandates that these issues be investigated and addressed during the preoperative visit.

Patient Fears

Patient education about what to expect before, during, and after refractive surgery is essential to a successful outcome. Discussion of a patient's fears should be part of the preoperative assessment.

FEAR OF THE UNKNOWN It is human nature to avoid conditions that we do not understand or have limited information about. Refractive surgery often falls into this category and may be avoided for the following reasons.

- minimal understanding or knowledge about advancements in techniques
- lack of widely publicized or circulated high surgical success rates and lack of understanding about complication rates
- uninformed coworkers or unhappy postoperative refractive patients used as sources of information

FEAR OF SURGERY The general population fears surgery for several reasons.

- effects of general anesthesia (e.g., nausea, vomiting)
- possibility of technical or human error by the surgeon or staff
- death or disfigurement

POSTOPERATIVE FEARS As with other surgeries, patients often fear what life will be like after the procedure. Typical fears include the following.
• intense pain
• partial or total vision loss
• significant loss of central or peripheral vision
• permanent blindness

Ignorance

Lack of consumer education is probably the most significant reason why some otherwise qualified individuals do not seek refractive surgery. Misperceptions about the following topics contribute to their unwillingness to undergo surgery.

REFRACTIVE ERROR AND LEVEL OF CORRECTION Patients generally believe that their prescription is relatively severe because they cannot see without glasses. In reality the prescription is usually quite moderate.
• public misperceptions about possible ranges of correction (patients often believe that their refractive error is so severe that it cannot be surgically corrected)
• days of radial keratotomy and limited range of myopic correction
• hyperopia (patients often lack awareness about options because correction is often not required until later in life)
• presbyopia (see hyperopia)

TECHNOLOGICAL ADVANCES Technology has progressed significantly since radial keratotomy (RK) was first introduced in the United States in the late 1970s. Correctional techniques used by surgeons today utilize the excimer laser, corneal ring segments, or intraocular lenses (IOLs).

• hyperopic laser in situ keratomileusis (LASIK)
• hyperopic astigmatic LASIK
• cross-cylinder LASIK (for high and mixed astigmatism)
• multifocal IOLs
• intracorneal rings

APPLICABILITY OF MONOVISION Monovision correction by refractive surgery is a desirable alternative for two main reasons:
• its wide range of correction
• its applicability to patients of many ages

Cost

Many individuals who may be motivated to proceed with refractive surgery find the financial cost to be a prohibiting factor. Prospective patients may not be able to accurately compare the long-term costs of spectacle or contact-lens wear with the cost of refractive surgery.

FINANCING OPTIONS As with any other large-cost item, a patient may pay for refractive surgery using one of many financing options.
• personal loans
• low–interest-rate credit cards
• employer assistance programs (i.e., the patient's employer pays a portion of the cost or the company has negotiated a group discount with the provider)
• "flex-spending" accounts (with tax advantages in the United States)
• "cafeteria plans"
• insurance (possibly a future option for refractive surgery, but few examples currently exist)

Occupational Needs

Some occupations require glasses to be worn at all times while on the job or have visual-acuity restrictions.

- safety eyeglasses for protection
- perfect visual acuity (as for pilots)

Postoperative Patient Expectations

Even with a "perfect" refractive outcome, some patients may not be satisfied if surgery does not meet their expectations. Often, initial discussion about the patient's motivation sheds light on the person's expected postoperative outcome and determines the best method of patient education.

- counseling of type A personalities or patients who are acutely critical of their vision about possible visual adverse effects and sometimes even discouraging them from refractive surgery
- investigation of each patient's expectations and criteria for "good vision"
- demonstrations with eyeglasses or contacts essential for a successful "subjective" surgical outcome
- documentation that the patient is actively seeking refractive surgery (may prove valuable in postoperative discussions with patients who have unrealistic visual expectations)

OCULAR HISTORY

A patient's ocular history helps to identify any potential postoperative problems that may arise and allows for adjustment, postponement, or cancellation of the procedure in question if necessary.

Previous Trauma

- identification of any trauma in the cornea or other component of the visual axis that may alter corneal wound healing or potential visual outcome
- determination of condition, location, duration, and method of treatment (if possible)

Previous Ocular Surgery

The identification and evaluation of a patient's previous ocular surgery status is critical to the success of subsequent refractive surgery. Several situations must be considered.

- artificial alteration of the refractive index secondary to faulty assumptions or calculations based on the IOL, scleral buckle, or other retinal procedures
- increased risk of retinal complications after surgical intervention
- difficulty obtaining proper suction and resultant flap complications

Family History

A thorough family history may elucidate potential contraindications or concerns with refractive surgery and long-term visual prognosis. A positive history of any of the following warrants further careful ocular evaluation prior to surgical intervention.

- glaucoma
- past history of high intraocular pressure after topical steroid application
- corneal dystrophy or degeneration
- untreated retinal pathology (e.g., retinal holes, tears, or detachment)

Medical History

The preoperative systemic history should include questions related to several diseases and conditions, including pregnancy and lactation, that may affect a surgical candidate's suitability for surgery.

OCULAR DISEASES Presurgical assessment of refractive surgery candidates may reveal a history of several ocular diseases that precludes surgery or poses increased risk of intraoperative or postoperative complications.

- corneal dystrophy
- cataracts
- keratoconus

- iritis (must rule out preoperatively if visually symptomatic)
- herpetic infection
- corneal bacterial infection
- retinal disease

VASCULAR DISEASES Any vascular disease that compromises a person's ocular performance or health is a contraindication for refractive surgery. Some are listed here.
- hypertension
- diabetes mellitus
- clotting or other blood disorders

COLLAGEN VASCULAR DISEASES The severity of collagen vascular disease determines whether it needs to be evaluated before refractive surgery. Most patients with collagen vascular disease have very mild symptoms and use very little medication. If a patient is rheumatoid-factor positive and has severe collagen vascular disease, refractive procedures are contraindicated. Examples of collagen vascular disease are listed here.
- systemic lupus erythematous
- rheumatoid arthritis
- scleroderma
- fibromyalgia

INFLAMMATORY DISORDERS Inflammatory disorders, such as those listed below, should be controlled and stable prior to refractive surgery.
- multiple sclerosis
- hyperthyroidism
- Crohn's disease

INFECTIOUS DISEASES An active infectious disease is generally a contraindication for refractive surgery.
- viral
- bacterial
- fungal

Medications and Allergies
Certain drug therapies may be contraindicated or alter postoperative outcome in patients undergoing refractive surgery. Allergies must also be considered.
- isotretinoin (Accutane; Hoffmann-La Roche Inc., Nutley, NJ) [contraindicated in potential photorefractive keratectomy (PRK) patients because of increased risk of PRK haze]
- sumatriptin (increased risk for epithelial defects after refractive surgery)
- antimetabolites and antirheumatic drugs (prolong or retard wound healing after refractive surgery)
- topical or systemic allergies to metals, latex, or laser gases

Prior Corrective Lenses
The patient's refractive history provides data that enables the surgeon to utilize the surgical correction that will provide the best vision over the patient's lifetime.
- frequency of previous visual exams
- refractive stability over the last few years
- frequency of and reason for changes in spectacle or contact lens prescription
- acceptance and adaptability of various near-correction options
- problems wearing eyeglasses or contact lenses (e.g., discomfort and intolerance)
- frequency and duration of contact lens wear (typical schedule)
- contact lens type (e.g., rigid gas permeable, hydrogel, polymethyl methacrylate)
- acceptance of monovision or bifocal contact-lens correction

INFORMED CONSENT

Informed consent is an essential part of any medical procedure, and its importance cannot be overemphasized. An estimated 1 in 1000 refractive surgery patients eventually sue their eyecare physician. Given the malpractice risks and subjective nature of many postoperative complaints, informed consent educates the patient about realistic expectations for the procedural outcome as well as the potential risks involved. Failure to obtain consent is an invitation to legal liability.

Fundamentals
- disclosure of risks and benefits to patient
- patient comprehension of the information provided
- voluntary submission by patient to surgery

Key Components
- physician-patient communication
  - may not be replaced by another form of consent prior to the procedure (e.g., videotapes, CDs, or staff-directed consent)
  - allows patient to ask any unanswered questions
- detailed educational description of diagnosis and proposed procedure
- list of potential benefits (based on recent outcome data so that patients can form realistic expectations)
- outline of alternative procedures
  - lists descriptions of alternatives required by many states
  - provides patient with the understanding that if he or she chooses to forgo refractive surgery, glasses and contact lenses continue to be effective
- outline of all risks, regardless of severity
  - educates the patient about all the risks of refractive procedures, even if risk is low
  - reminds patient that all procedures have risks and reminds the patient about the possibility of complications
    - includes risk for loss of best-corrected visual acuity (BCVA) (10–15% of eyes lose one line of BCVA and 2–5% of eyes may lose two or more lines of BCVA, an important risk to review with pilots and other regulated professions that require 20/20 BCVA)
    - mentions rare risk for blindness (should be described to emphasize the seriousness of the procedure)
    - does not necessarily mention unforeseeable, remote, or commonly known complications (such as death, although some surgeons have suggested that it should be mentioned)
- no guarantee of results (patients often ask for one and may be dissatisfied with results that are quite successful but do not necessarily match the patient's preoperative expectations; notification of no guaranteed results is included in the written consent form)
- possibility that additional procedures may be necessary
  - informs patient that enhancement procedures are often required for corneal refractive procedures
  - describes the potential need for additional procedures in order to provide the best uncorrected visual acuity (UCVA)
- potential need for glasses or contact lenses after procedure
  - states that the aim of refractive surgery is the *reduction* of dependence on glasses or contact lenses but not necessarily the *elimination* of the need for corrective lenses
  - informs presbyopic patients that they still may require glasses for reading
- jurisdiction of legal action
  - indicates that any potential legal proceeding would occur in the region of the refractive center rather than the home state or province of the patient (particu-

larly relevant if the patient travels to another country, such as Canada)
- state-specific requirements (forms should be reviewed to ensure that any state-specific requirements are included)

Special Considerations
- Review any new developments in complications or technology that apply to refractive surgery.
- Obtain U.S. Food and Drug Administration disclosure for any procedures that have not been approved.
- Obtain investigational device exception disclosure for device exceptions.
- Send the consent form to the patient at least 24 hours before the procedure to allow the patient to assimilate the information.
- Obtain consent for bilateral procedures.
- Reference the patient to optometric follow-up.
- Instruct patients to write out key concepts to demonstrate that they understand them (e.g., "I understand that there are no guarantees").
- Disclose all fees, including comanagement fees.

- The doctor also needs to sign the consent and include notes about any unique aspects of the case.

Suggested Readings

LASIK model consent form. American Society of Cataract and Refractive Surgery (member resource material). 2000; http://www.ascrs.org

Machat JJ. Preoperative myopic and hyperopic LASIK evaluation. In: Machat JJ, Slade SD, Probst LE, eds. *The Art of LASIK*. Thorofare, NJ: Slack Inc.; 2000:127–128.

O'Brart DPS. Preoperative considerations of corneal topography. In: Wu H, Steiner R, Slade S, Thompson V, eds. *Refractive Surgery*. New York: Thieme; 1999:79–88.

Portman R. Informed consent: questions and answers? *EyeWorld*. November 1999 (http://www.eyeworld.org).

Thompson VM, Wallin D. Patient selection and preoperative considerations. In: Wu H, Steiner R, Slade S, Thompson V, eds. *Refractive Surgery*. New York: Thieme; 1999:41–52.

CHAPTER 5

General Ocular Evaluation

Andrea D. Border, John F. Doane, Scot Morris, and James A. Denning

CHAPTER CONTENTS

VISUAL ACUITY ASSESSMENT

Methods

• Measure uncorrected distance, near, monocular, and binocular visual acuity. (Fig. 5–1).
• Measure best corrected visual acuity (BCVA) for distance, near, monocular, and binocular vision with patient wearing prescribed spectacles or contact lenses (if applicable).
• Measure and document acuity preoperatively and at all postoperative evaluations for statistical assessment, progression analysis, and medicolegal documentation.
• Carefully educate patients with reduced acuity because of pathology or amblyopia

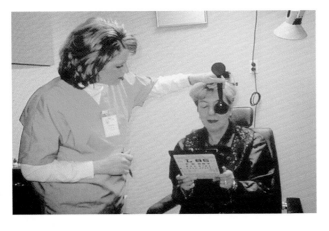

Figure 5–1 Pre- and post-operative near-vision acuity should be taken for each eye and both eyes together.

that refractive surgery probably will not improve their BCVA.

Postoperative Patient Management
- Show documentation of a patient's pre-operative uncorrected visual acuity to help provide perspective if he or she is unhappy with the postoperative result.
- Compare a patient's pre- and postoperative BCVA to reassure the patient that his or her best corrected vision has not changed.
- Extreme myopes may have decreased acuity with spectacle correction because high-power minus lenses minify the size of objects in the spectacle plane.
- Wearers of hard or soft contact lenses may suffer decreased acuity because of poor-fitting lenses or undesirable tear film/contact lens interactions.
- Refractive surgery may improve acuity compared with spectacles or contact lenses but is not guaranteed.

EYE DOMINANCE TESTING

Indications
- manifest refraction binocular balance testing [the dominant eye is left with "clearer" vision when equal balance unobtainable for both eyes (see Chapter 6)]
- crucial for surgically created monovision (the dominant eye is almost always corrected for distance vision, and the nondominant eye is targeted for near or intermediate vision)
- confirmation or identification of a patient's dominant eye

Methods
- Ask the patient which eye he or she uses to look through a telescope or focus a camera (identified eye usually dominant).
- Perform some or all of the specific methods discussed below.

Pointing
The use of pointing to determine a patient's dominant eye is simple but obtained results may be unreliable.

Methods
- Instruct the patient to leave both eyes open and point at a distant object using an index finger and with the arm fully extended.
- If the object becomes displaced relative to the finger when the patient closes one eye, then the patient closed the dominant eye, but if the object did not become displaced, then the closed eye is nondominant.
- Repeat this test to confirm results.

Framing
The framing method of determining a patient's dominant eye is simple to perform but may provide ambiguous results.

Methods
- A patient uses both hands (thumbs and index fingers) to create a triangle-shaped "frame" around a readily identifiable, small, distant object (Fig. 5–2A).
- With arms fully extended and both eyes open, the patient frames the object and then brings both hands toward the face moderately quickly, keeping both eyes open with the distant object sighted and in focus the entire time (Fig. 5–2B). (The patient should frame the dominant eye.)
- If the patient cannot perform this task without seeing the distant object as "double," then the patient may be partially or totally *ambiocular* (i.e., without a strongly dominant eye).
- Instruct the patient to repeat the procedure to confirm results.

Hole Card
This test uses the same principle as the framing method but may also provide ambiguous results.

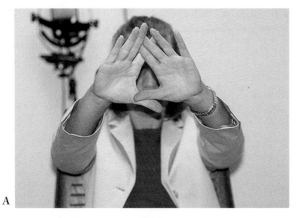

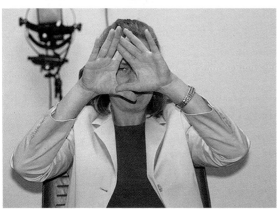

Figure 5–2 (A) The patient "frames" a distance target with both hands. (B) The patient should select (frame) the dominant eye.

A

B

Methods
- Create the hole card by punching a hole in the center of a small, square piece of paper (about the size of a prescription pad).
- Instruct the patient to hold the card with both hands and with arms extended.
- Ask the patient to sight a small, designated, distant object through the hole in the card with both eyes open.
- Ask the patient to bring the hole card swiftly back toward his or her face, keeping the object in focus and leaving both eyes open. (The patient should bring the hole card back to the dominant eye.)
- If the patient cannot sight the object through the hole without seeing "double,"

the patient may be partially or totally ambiocular.
- Repeat this test several times to confirm the dominant eye.

Four Base Out Test
The pointing, framing, and hole card tests may yield ambiguous results, but the four base out (BO) test provides definitive results.

Methods
- Place a four prism diopter lens BO over the patient's suspected dominant eye while the patient fixates with both eyes on a distant object (Fig. 5–3).

REFRACTIVE SURGERY: A COLOR SYNOPSIS

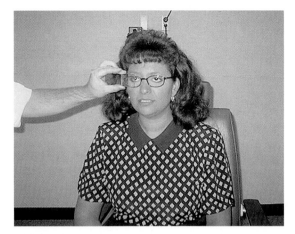

Figure 5–3 The examiner places a four-prism diopter lens BO over the patient's suspected dominant eye as the patient fixates on a distant target.

○ If this is truly the patient's dominant eye, the examiner should notice a "shift" in the patient's opposite (nondominant) eye as it attempts to re-fixate.

• Next, place the 4^Δ BO prism over the suspected nondominant eye with the patient fixating on the same distant object.

○ If this is truly the patient's nondominant eye, the examiner should note little to no eye shift in the opposite (dominant) eye.

○ If the examiner has difficulty detecting eye shift versus no eye shift when presenting the prism to either eye, try increasing the prism amount to elicit a more substantial reaction.

• If the 4^Δ BO test and the other eye dominance tests yield conflicting results, then consider the patient to be ambiocular. (Generally, ambiocular patients do not accept monovision well and should be considered very cautiously as monovision candidates.)

MONOVISION CONSIDERATIONS

Preoperative Considerations
• the patient's personality, age, hobbies, and goals for refractive surgery

• determination of monovision target power (allows a patient adequate near/intermediate vision while maintaining acceptable distance vision)

• testing of patients who use computers regularly by using the patient's habitual computer font size and working distance at a computer terminal

• realistic patient expectations about surgical results

• ambiocular patients (of 1 in 10 patients in general population unable to accept any level of monovision, most are difficult to measure and quantify; see Eye Dominance Testing)

• patient preference of the dominant eye for near vision (should be attempted only with careful trials and documentation and after performing a trial run of monovision with contact lenses)

• previous monovision failure

○ possible success with surgical monovision for patients with previously unsuccessful monovision contact lenses (may have been caused by dry eyes, poor lens fit, inaccurate lens powers, or improper eye selection)

○ consider cautiously as surgical candidates until proven otherwise

○ requires preoperative trial frames for motivated patients

- patient education
  - discussion of advantages and compromises of monovision with all presbyopic patients and those older than 40 years, the average age of onset for presbyopia (highly motivated patients <40 years old may be considered if thoroughly educated and intent on undergoing the procedure)
  - the possible reversibility of monovision with enhancement surgery if monovision unacceptable [most applicable for radial keratotomy (RK), photorefractive radial keratectomy (PRK), and laser in situ keratomileusis (LASIK) myopic candidates who are intentionally undercorrected in one eye to create monovision]
  - notification of the possible postoperative adjustment period that lasts from one to several weeks and may be disorienting
  - advantages (lifelong decreased or eliminated dependence on spectacles for near and intermediate tasks)
  - disadvantages (possible scotopic halos and glare, compromised depth perception in dim lighting that may be alleviated by thin night-driving eyeglasses)
- documentation of the discussion about monovision
  - the patient's decision for or against monovision
  - the patient's understanding of possible consequences of his or her choice (e.g., possibility of increased night glare vs. need for reading glasses)

Monovision Trial Framing
Indications
- identification of poor monovision candidates before surgically creating monovision (Fig. 5–4)
- determination of monovision target powers

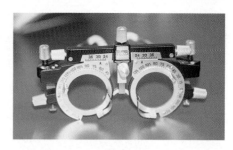

Figure 5–4 The trial frame is set up with the patient's manifest refraction results for each eye, and an occluder lens is then placed over the patient's dominant eye. The examiner should place a plus power lens appropriate for the patient's age and visual goals over the patient's nondominant eye.

Methods
- Place the patient's manifest refraction result for each eye in the trial frame.
- Place an occluder lens in the trial frame over the patient's dominant eye (see Eye Dominance Testing for methods).
- Instruct the patient to look at a near vision card, and place a plus lens (for monovision) over the unoccluded eye.
- Select the power of the plus lens based on the patient's age (from +1.00 D at 40 years of age to +2.00 D at 55 years of age) and visual goals (e.g., small near tasks like threading a needle or general intermediate tasks such as seeing a computer).
- After acknowledging the patient's ability to see the near card, remove the occluder lens from the trial frame over the patient's dominant eye to allow the patient to see binocularly in monovision
  - The patient initially may report ghosting or doubling of the near letters with binocular monovision in the trial frame (often occurs if the optical center is off in the trial frame lenses).
  - Instruct the patient to shift the near card slightly to attempt to remove the ghosting.

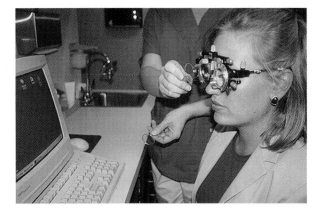

Figure 5–5 After visual acuities are taken at distance and near with the tentative monovision target, the technician can walk with the patient to allow visualization of various distances in monovision. This patient desires clear computer vision, and the technician is trying various monovision powers to achieve the best focus for the patient at a computer terminal.

- Next, allow the patient to experience monovision at various distances with the trial frame by having the patient walk around with a technician.
- Try various monovision target powers with the patient (Fig. 5–5).
  - For example, if a 46-year-old patient has an initial monovision target of +1.50 D but does not see a computer screen well with this lens, the technician should try a target of +1.00 D at the computer).
  - If more acceptable to the patient and agreeable with the patient's goals, adjust the target.
- If a patient chronically experiences significant ghosting of near letters or experiences outright diplopia or nausea that does not subside, the patient will probably not tolerate monovision.
- Single-vision soft contact lenses (for patients who have essentially spherical refractive errors) are an easy, inexpensive way to allow refractive surgery candidates to experience monovision in their own home or work environment.

PUPILLOMETRY

Indications
- identification of patients with physiologically large pupils

- may warrant patient counseling about possible irreversible night-glare symptoms after RK or laser refractive surgery procedures
  - may have problematic glare symptoms because of small clear, corneal optical zones created by incisions during surgery (specifically RK)
  - may experience induction of glare, halos, or "star bursting" with laser ablation zone sizes smaller than scotopic pupil sizes (with PRK and LASIK)
- determination of likelihood of patient complaints (few complain about nocturnal vision 3 months postoperatively although occasionally a patient with normal or smaller than average pupils complains of poor night vision associated with the procedure, even when all objective tests are within normal limits)

Pupil Card
This is probably the easiest and least expensive method for evaluating pupil size but may be less accurate than other methods.

Methods
- Simply line up semicircles (usually ranging from 1.0 to 10.0 mm in increments of 1.0 mm) at the vertical midpoint of the patient's pupil and determine which semicircle on the card best represents the patient's pupil size (Fig. 5–6).

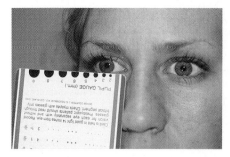

Figure 5–6 Pupil size is measured with a pupil card in photopic and mesopic conditions to determine minimum and maximum physiologic pupil size in a patient.

• Record corresponding measurements from the pupil card in both photopic (light) and mesopic (dim) conditions.

Holladay-Godwin Pupil Gauge

This gauge (American Surgical Instrument Corporation, Westmont, IL) was designed to make pupil measurement simple and accurate.

Methods

• Use this gauge in the same manner as the pupil card.
• Measure pupil sizes larger than 0.5 mm in scotopic and mesopic conditions by comparing actual pupil size with the full circles and semicircles on the gauge (from 1.0 to 10.0 mm in increments of 0.5 mm) (Fig. 5–7A).

Colvard Pupillometer

This hand-held, battery-operated pupillometer from Oasis (Glendora, CA) preoperatively evaluates and measures the scotopic and photopic pupil size. It allows accurate visualization of the pupil in a darkened examination room by incorporating light amplification technology for accurate scotopic measurements (Fig. 5–7B).

SLIT-LAMP EXAMINATION

Indications

• preoperative identification of pterygium (ideally, elimination of it prior to any corneal surgery)
• identification of corneal neovascularization or pannus (significant intraoperative bleeding may occur during corneal procedures with either of these)
• identification of corneal endothelial pigment spindles (may indicate future or current pigment dispersion, glaucoma)
• preoperative documentation of intraocular pressure (IOP) (future readings will be lower than preoperative values by approximately 1.5 mmHg/100 μm of ablated tissue for laser procedures during which significant corneal tissue is removed)
• identification of inactive corneal opacities and/or scars and assessment of their impact on visual acuity (Fig. 5–8; see Chapter 3)

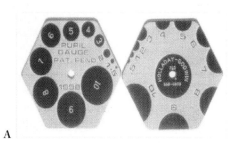 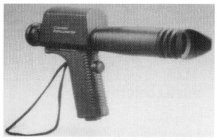

A   B

Figure 5–7 (A) The Holladay-Godwin pupil gauge. (B) The Colvard pupil gauge.

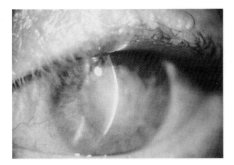

Figure 5–8 Central corneal scars or opacities must be evaluated for their impact on visual acuity.

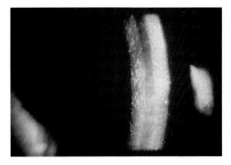

Figure 5–9 Severe corneal gutatta seen in retroillumination. This patient has a reduced endothelial cell count shown by specular microscopy.

- identification of dry eye or keratoconjunctivitis sicca (if severe, then may be *contraindications* for corneal surgery)
- recognition of anterior basement membrane dystrophy (may complicate LASIK procedures intraoperatively or delay visual recovery with any refractive surgery procedure) (see Chapter 3)

Relative Contraindications for Surgery
- corneal disease
- prior corneal surgery
- specific orbit configurations
- abnormal eyelid closure (lagophthalmos) because of increased risk for delayed corneal healing
- poorly healed corneal scars (may ablate more easily than surrounding tissue)
- signs of prior herpes simplex or zoster keratitis (because of reduced corneal sensitivity and potential for reactivation of infection)

Absolute Contraindications for Surgery
- endothelial dystrophies (such as Fuchs' dystrophy or severe gutatta with a total cell count <1500) (Fig. 5–9; see Chapter 3)
  - increased risk for future corneal edema and decompensation (bullous keratopathy)
  - particularly worrisome with clear lens extraction refractive surgery (associated with a 4–8% cell loss during the procedure)
- any active anterior segment infectious or inflammatory process (must be completely resolved preoperatively)
- keratoconus with or without Vogt's stria or Fleischer's ring (Fig. 5–10) (for any corneal refractive surgical procedure)

FUNDUS EXAMINATION

Indications
- identification and discussion of macular pathology such as pathological myopic degeneration, age-related macular

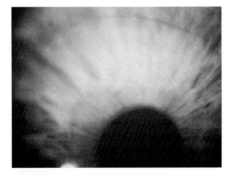

Figure 5–10 Fleischer's ring seen around the base of the cone in a patient with keratoconus.

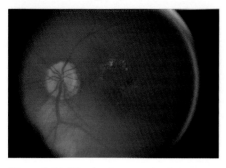

Figure 5–11 Macular degeneration has not yet affected visual acuity in this patient.

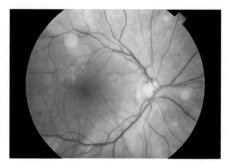

Figure 5–12 Severe glaucomatous damage has already occurred in this optic nerve, but central visual acuity is not yet affected in this patient.

degeneration, or diabetic retinopathy (Fig. 5–11) (discussion with patient warranted if pathology has already affected visual function because refractive surgery will not increase the patient's BCVA)
• identification of patients with prior vitreoretinal, cataract, or strabismus surgery (may complicate refractive surgical procedures such as LASIK or clear lens extraction)
• identification of significant vitreal syneresis or lattice degeneration associated with traction or holes (may complicate LASIK or clear lens extraction refractive surgical procedures)
• identification of severe glaucoma or other optic nerve disorders (consider on a case-by-case basis) (Fig. 5–12)
  ○ IOP rises transiently during LASIK surgery
  ○ poor long-term visual prognoses of severe glaucoma with any refractive surgical procedure
• identification of retinitis pigmentosa (consider on a case-by-case basis with emphasis on patient counseling)

  ○ aggravation of the associated attenuated vasculature and optic nerve changes because of marked transient rise in IOP during LASIK
  ○ inhibition of night vision in patients with retinitis pigmentosa after other refractive surgical procedures, including LASIK
• identification and evaluation of posterior staphyloma using ultrasonography particularly when considering clear lens extraction (see Chapter 7)

Suggested Readings

Assil KK, Schanzlin DJ. *Radial and Astigmatic Keratotomy: A Complete Handbook.* St. Louis: Poole Press; 1994.

Carlson NB, Kurtz D, Heath DA, Hines C. *Clinical Procedures for Ocular Examination.* Norwalk, CT: Appleton & Lange; 1990.

Machat JJ, Slade SG, Probst LE. *The Art of LASIK.* 2nd ed. Thorofare, NJ: Slack Inc.; 1999.

CHAPTER 6

Evaluation of Refractive Error and Pre- and Postoperative Data

Andrea D. Border, John F. Doane, Scot Morris, and James A. Denning

CHAPTER CONTENTS

Retinoscopy

Binocular Fog Manifest Refraction

Binocular Balancing

Trial Frame Refraction

Cycloplegic Retinoscopy and Refraction

Keratometry

Computerized Corneal Topography

Keratoscopy

Pachymetry

Specular Microscopy

Ultrasonic Scanning

High-Frequency Anterior Segment Ultrasound Biomicroscopy

Contrast Sensitivity Testing

Suggested Readings

Before undergoing refractive surgery, a candidate's refractive error and other preoperative data, such as that from pachymetry and topography, must be evaluated to ensure consistent and accurate surgical results. Likewise, postoperative data need to be evaluated to decrease the likelihood of complications and to increase the possibility of favorable surgical results. Autorefraction may provide a useful starting point for baseline preoperative refraction but should not be used for postoperative testing because it often gives erroneous results (Fig. 6–1).

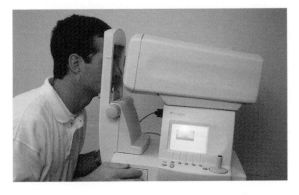

Figure 6–1 The autorefractor by Humphrey gives spectacle refractive error and K values.

RETINOSCOPY

Indications
• starting point for determination of a patient's manifest refractive error (required of all refractive surgery candidates)

Methods
• Enter the correct distance pupil diameter into the phoropter.
• Place the phoropter in front of the patient, making sure it is level with the patient's head.
• Relax accommodation by "fogging" the patient with plus-power lenses, placing a moderate amount of spherical plus power over the patient's habitual prescription into the phoropter (+1.50 to +2.00 D).
• Present the 20/60 line of Snellen's chart to each individual eye. (If the line is too blurry to read with either eye, the patient is adequately fogged.)
• Present a 20/400 distance target (e.g., the "E" from Snellen's chart) to the patient for fixation using both eyes (OU).
• Perform retinoscopy one eye at a time while OU are unoccluded.
• Do not remove the retinoscopic working-distance lenses (usually +1.50 D) from the phoropter (can trigger patient accommodation).
• Adjust the working-distance lenses accordingly if you perform retinoscopy particularly close to or far from the phoropter.
• Record the retinoscopic findings for comparison with manifest refraction results.
• Note the retinoscopic reflex (should be bright and clear, not dull).
• Note any "scissoring" of the reflex motion (a hallmark sign of keratoconus).
• Proceed directly to binocular fog manifest refraction.

BINOCULAR FOG MANIFEST REFRACTION

Myopia
• determination of refractive error with a phoropter after retinoscopy (for all patients)

Methods
• Follow these steps carefully to reduce chances of over-minus refractive results.
• Fog with plus-power lenses to relax accommodation. [Initially, fog the right eye (OD) by +1.50 D and the left (OS) by +3.00 D.]
• Note that myopes can easily accept too much minus power for their manifest refraction endpoint if not properly fogged (results in postoperative overcorrection).
• If retinoscopy immediately preceded manifest refraction, OD should already be fogged and so simply add another +1.50 D over OS to complete the initial fogging (see section on Retinoscopy).
• With both of the patient's eyes unoccluded, present the isolated 20/60 line from Snellen's chart.
• Inform the patient that vision for OU should be fuzzy, with vision for the left eye being extremely fuzzy. (Patients should guess at letters during the exam if unsure).
• Emphasize the importance of keeping OU open for the duration of testing.
• Begin binocular fog manifest refraction for the right eye (OD) by *slowly* stepping down the patient from plus-sphere power while presenting successively smaller isolated acuity lines from Snellen's visual acuity chart.
  ○ Ask the patient to read the acuity line that is presented with each 0.25 D decrease in plus-sphere power.

- Stop decreasing plus-sphere power when the patient is able to *just see* the smallest achievable acuity line without noticing any minification of the letters.
- Refine the cylinder amount and axis OD using the phoropter's Jackson crossed cylinder (JCC) and one line *larger* than the patient's smallest achievable acuity line as the target.
- Fog OD again with enough plus power to blur the 20/50 line.
  - Slowly step the patient out of plus power, asking the patient if the final step-down lenses make the target line clearer and easier to read or just smaller and darker (minified).
  - If the patient notices minification of the letters but acuity does not improve, then the patient is probably over-minused in power. This is the monocular endpoint for OD. [Mild over-minus power (−0.25 to −1.00 D) can make distance targets appear subjectively "darker" and, therefore, falsely "clearer" to the patient.]
- After this final step down from plus-sphere power, isolate the line of the patient's best corrected visual acuity (BCVA).
- Double check that the monocular endpoint is correct by adding two or three "clicks" of plus-sphere power (+0.50 to +0.75 D) over OD. (The patient should require no more than 0.50 to 0.75 D of plus power to blur out the BCVA line; if more plus power is required, then the patient is over minused.)
- After reaching the monocular *endpoint* for OD (see above), keep the right eye unoccluded and fog it by +3.00 D.
- Decrease plus-sphere power in OS until he or she is just able to see the 20/60 line of Snellen's chart.
- Repeat the steps used for OD for OS.
- After reaching the manifest refraction monocular endpoint for both OD and OS, balance the patient for binocular accommodation (see page 48 for balance techniques).

Hyperopia
Indications
- See section on myopia for indications.

Methods
- The procedure for binocular fog manifest refraction of hyperopes is identical to that for myopes.
- Follow the steps for myopic binocular fog manifest refraction carefully to reduce the chance of underestimating the true amount of plus power of the refraction. (Hyperopes may not accept full plus power on the manifest refraction endpoint if they are not properly fogged, and even with proper fogging, they still may not accept the full amount of plus power discovered on retinoscopic evaluation (i.e., latent hyperopia.)
- Proceed to a cycloplegic examination to reveal the actual amount of hyperopia for patients with suspected latent hyperopia.

Astigmatism
Indications
- to confirm the amount of astigmatism found with retinoscopy, keratometry, and corneal topography (usually agrees)
  - Compensation for over-minus sphere power by approximately twice the amount of plus cylinder power is a relatively common error found in spectacle prescriptions.
  - For example, if a patient's true prescription is $-6.00 + 2.00 \times 090$, he or she may actually have an inaccurate prescription of $-7.00 + 4.00 \times 090$ (avoid by making sure that retinoscopy results correspond with manifest refraction results).

- to quantify the amount of astigmatism in infrequent cases of almost total noncorneal (i.e., lenticular or ocular) astigmatism (usually much greater than that found on keratometry or corneal topography)
- to evaluate the consistency of the corneal topographical cylinder with reconstruction of the sphero-cylindrical manifest refraction (Fig. 6–2) in the infrequent cases of nonorthogonal astigmatism (i.e., the two steep meridians differ by more than 180 degrees)

Methods
- The procedure for astigmatic binocular fog manifest refraction is exactly the same as that described for myopic-binocular fog manifest refraction.
- If you cannot reconcile retinoscopic results with manifest refraction results, perform a cycloplegic retinoscopy and manifest refraction.

BINOCULAR BALANCING

Indications
- mandatory matching of accommodative stimulus for OU for all surgical candidates who may have some accommodative ability in reserve (i.e., patients younger than 60 years of age)
- corroboration of initial results [If you strictly followed the steps for binocular fog manifest refraction (see page 46), most patients are already balanced for accommodation.

Methods
- Determine the patient's dominant eye before attempting binocular balance (see Chapter 5 for eye dominance testing).
- Generally perform balance techniques with a phoropter after arriving at the monocular endpoints for binocular fog manifest refraction.

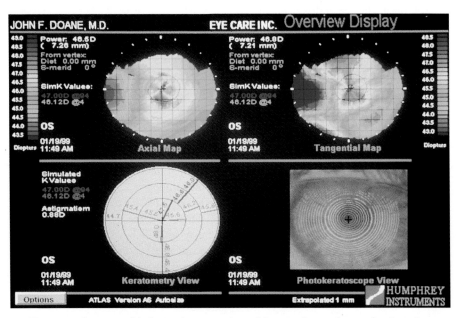

Figure 6–2 A topographical map shows a patient with nonorthogonal corneal astigmatism.

• If a patient cannot be equally balanced by any method, leave the dominant eye with clearer vision. (See Chapter 5 for tests to determine eye dominance.)

Fogged Prism Disassociated Balance

Methods

• Make sure both of the patient's eyes are open behind the phoropter.
• Fog each eye to slightly over the monocular endpoint obtained with binocular fog manifest refraction by +0.75 D sphere power (Fig. 6–3).
• Isolate one or two acuity lines worse than the patient's BCVA line on the projected distance chart.
• Place three prism diopters base down (BD) over OD and three base up (BU) over OS using the phoropter's rotary (Risley's) prisms.
• Inform the patient that he or she should see two "fuzzy" lines of letters, one above the other.
  ◦ If the patient sees only one line, try increasing the vertical prism to four to

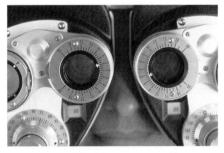

Figure 6–3 This patient has been fogged by +0.75 D over the manifest refraction result for OU for fogged prism disassociated balancing. To disassociate the patient's eyes, three prism diopters BD have been placed over OD and three prism diopters BU have been placed over OS using the Risley's prisms of the phoropter.

six prism diopters over each eye and make sure OU are open.
• If OU are open but the patient still sees only one line, abandon this balance procedure for one of the others described in this section.
• Instruct the patient to look at both lines with OU and report if one line looks clearer or if both lines appear *equally fuzzy.* (If equally fuzzy initially, then the patient is already balanced and the procedure is complete.)
• Add +0.25 D sphere power to the eye that sees the clearer line (i.e., make it blurrier). [If the lower line is clearer (the one seen by OS) then add +0.25 D to OS.]
• Ask the patient again if both lines are equally blurry.
• If not, ask the patient again which line is clearer and add +0.25 D to the eye seeing the clearer line.
• The endpoint is reached when the patient reports that both lines are equally clear or nearly equally clear. (If the patient cannot decide which line is clearest, then the patient cannot be balanced and you should leave the patient's dominant eye clearer by 0.25 D.)
• After achieving the endpoint, remove the prisms and step down the patient from plus-sphere power until the patient can read the BCVA line sharply without noticing any binocular minification of the letters.
• Record the resulting numbers for each eye as the patient's manifest refraction.

Red-Green Prism Disassociated Duochrome Balance

Indications

• an alternative to the fogged prism disassociated balance procedure. (With this method, accommodation is uncontrolled and over minus results are possible because the patient is not fogged during testing.)

- the only way to balance a patient with amblyopia (individually balances each eye under equal conditions simultaneously; each eye has a different BCVA with eyeglasses)

Methods
- Unocclude OU behind the phoropter.
- Isolate one line on Snellen's chart that is larger than the patient's BCVA line.
- Do not fog either eye.
- Cover the isolated line with the red-green filter.
- Using the phoropter's Risley's prisms, place three prism diopters BD over OD, and three BU over OS.
- Inform the patient that he or she should see two lines, one above the other.
  - If the patient sees only one line, make sure OU are open.
  - If patient's eyes are both open, increase the vertical prism to 4 or 6 D over each eye.
  - If the patient still does not see two lines, invert the prisms (i.e., place BU over OD and BD over OS).
  - If the patient *still* cannot see two lines, abandon the procedure for one that does not involve prism disassociation, such as fogged alternate cover balancing.
- Instruct the patient to look at the upper line only (the one seen by OD) while keeping OU open.
  - Tell the patient to look from the green side to the red side and then back to the green side.
  - Ask which side looks sharper and clearer or if both sides look equally clear.
  - If the green side is clearer, add +0.25 D to OD only; if the red side is clearer, add −0.25 D to OD.
  - If both the red and green sides look equally clear initially, proceed to balancing OS (i.e., direct the patient to look at the lower line).

- The *endpoint* for OD is achieved when both sides appear equally clear. (If both sides are not equally clear and the patient cannot decide which one is clearer, leave the green side clearer than the red side by 0.25 D.)
- Direct the patient's attention to the lower line (the one seen by OS), and repeat the steps described for OD using the same endpoint criterion.
- If a patient always chooses the same side (red or green) as clearer regardless of which lens is presented, abandon the duochrome test for another balancing method.
- Record the endpoints for OD/OS as the manifest refraction results.

Fogged Alternate Cover Balance
Indications
- an alternative to fogged prism disassociated and red-green prism disassociated duochrome balance methods for patients unresponsive to those tests

Methods
- Fog each eye +0.75 D sphere power over the endpoint of binocular fog manifest refraction behind the phoropter.
- Isolate one or two acuity lines worse than the patient's BCVA line on Snellen's acuity chart.
- Instruct the patient to keep OU open during testing.
- Inform the patient that he or she should see one "fuzzy" line.
- Alternately cover the viewing holes in the phoropter with a cover paddle for each eye (Fig. 6–4).
- Cover and uncover each eye a few times and ask the patient to notice if one line appears clearer or if OU appear to have equally blurry vision.
  - If one eye appears to have clearer vision, add +0.25 D sphere power over that eye only.

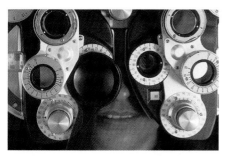

Figure 6–4 This patient has been fogged by +0.75 D OU over the manifest refraction for fogged alternate cover binocular balancing. A cover paddle alternately covers each eye behind the phoropter.

   ◦ Continue alternately covering the eyes and adding +0.25 D sphere power until the lines are equally blurry, the *endpoint* of the test.
   ◦ If unable to achieve equality, leave the patient's dominant eye clearer but leave the nondominant eye as clear as possible.
   ◦ If OU appear equally blurry initially, then the patient is already balanced and further balance testing is unnecessary.
- After achieving the endpoint, step down the patient from plus sphere power (binocularly) until the BCVA line is clear and sharp but the patient notices no minification of letters.
- Record the resulting numbers for each eye as the patient's manifest refraction.

TRIAL FRAME REFRACTION

Indications
- "fine tuning" of the results of binocular fog manifest refraction and binocular balance (see pages 46 and 48, respectively) when a patient's spherical equivalent refractive error is more than 4.00 D
- confirmation of results from binocular fog manifest refraction for patients with accommodative instability (Vertex distance can be held constant and peripheral fusion cues are left intact in a trial frame although for patients with very deep-set or proptotic eyes, a trial frame may not achieve the average vertex distance.)
- another option for retinoscopy and binocular fog manifest refraction on patients who are unable to sit behind a phoropter
- generally more accurate refinement of refraction than the phoropter because you can control vertex distance and leave peripheral fusion locks intact

Methods
- Clean trial lenses with a soft, clean lens cloth.
- Place a combination of spherical and cylindrical trial lenses into the trial frame that equal the balanced manifest refraction results for each eye.
   ◦ Place the sphere lens in the single well on the back side of the trial frame.
   ◦ Place any cylinder lens on the correct axis in the first (closest to the eye) well on the front of the trial frame.
   ◦ Lock the cylinder axis in place with the axis lock knob.
   ◦ Place any other necessary sphere lenses to equal the manifest refraction result in the middle well on the front side of the trial frame.
- Place an occluder lens in the last well on the front side of the trial frame over the patient's nondominant eye (Fig. 6–5). (See Chapter 5 for tests to determine eye dominance.)
- Place the trial frame on the patient and adjust it for the correct temple length to the correct vertex distance, frame height (via nose pad adjustment knob), pantoscopic tilt, and interpupillary distance.
- Inform the patient that he or she can see out of only one eye because an occluder is in place over the nondominant eye.

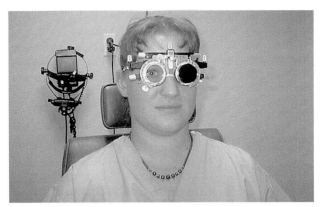

Figure 6–5 The trial frame is prepared for trial frame refraction with lenses that equal the patient's manifest refraction results obtained with the phoropter. An occluder lens is placed over the patient's nondominant eye.

- Measure the vertex distance with a distometer (Fig. 6–6). (For prescriptions >4.00 D, vertex distance becomes significant with respect to power at the cornea.)
  - Try to keep a consistent vertex distance between patients to minimize confusion of vertex distance conversions. (Excimer lasers allow for a set vertex distance of 12.5 mm.)
- If you cannot obtain a normal vertex distance, note the actual vertex distance and adjust for power accordingly when necessary. (Vertex distance affects a patient's acceptance of power for distance vision in

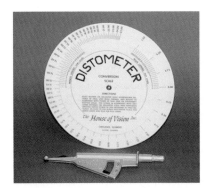

Figure 6–6 A distometer is used to measure the distance between the patient's eye and the trial frame lens (vertex distance) and comes with a wheel chart for conversion from millimeters of vertex distance to diopters of power.

the trial frame: above average distance means a patient accepts too much minus power; below average distance indicates that a patient accepts too much plus power.)
- Show the patient his or her BCVA line from Snellen's acuity chart, and ask the patient to read that line using the unoccluded eye. (If the patient cannot read the line, be sure the sphere and cylinder powers and axis are correct and that the lenses are clean.)
- Refine the sphere power in the trial frame.
  - Present a +0.50 D sphere lens over the unoccluded eye and ask the patient if it makes the line clearer and easier to read, or more blurry.
  - If the line is more blurry, put the lens aside.
  - If the lens makes the letters clearer and easier to read, place a +0.25 D lens in the front well.
- Re-present the +0.50 D lens. (If the patient still sees more clearly with the lens, remove the +0.25 D lens and add the +0.50 D lens to the front well.)
- Present a +0.50 D lens a final time. (If the line is still clearer, then the manifest refraction results are probably wrong.)
- Next, present a −0.50 D sphere lens over the unoccluded eye, and ask the patient if it makes the line clearer and easier to read, or just smaller and darker (minified).

REFRACTIVE SURGERY: A COLOR SYNOPSIS

- If the line is just smaller and darker, put the lens aside.
- If the line is clearer and easier to read, add a −0.25 D sphere lens to the front well.
- Present the −0.50 D lens again. (If the patient still sees more clearly with the lens and does not notice minification of the letters, remove the −0.25 D lens and put the −0.50 D lens in the front well.)
- Present the −0.50 D lens a final time. (If the line is still clearer and not just smaller and darker, then the manifest refraction results are probably wrong.)
- Record the sphere power selected after performing these steps as the trial frame refraction sphere power.
- Refine the cylinder axis if the patient's astigmatism is more than 0.50 D.
  - Inform the patient that he or she will be refining the astigmatism axis.
  - Isolate one line worse than the patient's BCVA line on Snellen's acuity chart.
  - Guide the patient's corresponding hand (i.e., right hand for the right eye) to the cylinder axis adjustment knob on the trial frame.
  - Loosen the axis lock knob.
  - Instruct the patient to hold the adjustment knob between the thumb and forefinger and to look at the isolated line.
  - Tell the patient to slowly turn the knob forward and backward until the line becomes as clear as possible.
  - Patients with only 0.75 to 1.00 D of cylinder power may have a range of approximately 10 degrees where the letters appear to be equally clear. (In this case, tell the patient to stop turning the knob when in the approximate middle of the "clear range.")
  - If the patient has selected an axis that is significantly different (>5 degrees) than the manifest refraction axis, adjust the axis yourself between the manifest refraction and cylinder axes.
  - Ask the patient whether one or two is clearer as you stop at each axis.
- Record the selected axis as the trial frame refraction axis.
- Unocclude the other eye and place the occluder lens over the eye that has already been refined.
- Repeat the steps for refining sphere power and cylinder axis for the other eye.
- After refining OU, unocclude them and check the patient's visual acuity with OU on the Snellen's acuity chart.
- Record the power and axis in the trial frame for each eye as the trial frame refraction.
- These results should be consistent (within +0.50 or −0.50 D spherical equivalent power and within +0.10 or −10 degrees of cylinder axis) with retinoscopic and binocular fog manifest refraction results.
- If results are inconsistent, recheck the results or perform a cycloplegic examination.
- When refining the sphere power in the trial frame, always present plus lenses first to avoid an accommodative response from the patient.
- The spherical *endpoint* in the trial frame should be no more than ± −0.50 D from the manifest refraction endpoint; if further than this endpoint, the manifest refraction is probably wrong and should be reevaluated.
- You may refine cylinder *power* in the trial frame with a hand-held cylindrical lens, also known as a Jackson cross cylinder (JCC), that usually has ±0.25 D cylinder of power at ninety degrees (not usually necessary unless the cylinder power is questioned).

CYCLOPLEGIC RETINOSCOPY AND REFRACTION

Indications
- identification of suspected latent hyperopia or accommodative spasm

- evaluation of unexplainable acuity fluctuations during the refractive process (also can be explained by poor tear film)
- investigation of large inconsistencies among retinoscopic, binocular fog manifest refraction, and trial frame refraction results

Methods
- Diligent fogging techniques are unnecessary for cycloplegic retinoscopy and manifest refraction.
- Tropicamide (1%) (Mydriacil, Opticyl) is usually adequate when performing a cycloplegic examination on adult patients (Fig. 6–7)
  - In extreme cases of latent hyperopia or accommodative spasm, you may need to use stronger cycloplegic agents (cyclopentolate 0.5%).
  - Administer two drops of 1% tropicamide 10 minutes apart, and begin examination at least 20 minutes after administration of the last drop.
- For cyclopentolate, the maximum duration of action is longer so it is best to wait 40 to 60 minutes before proceeding with the refractive examination.

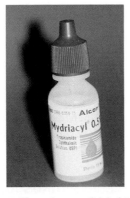

Figure 6–7 Two drops of Mydriacyl 1% (tropicamide), administered 10 minutes apart, is generally considered adequate for cycloplegic refraction of an adult patient.

- In all cases, perform retinoscopy for a cycloplegic examination before manifest refraction behind the phoropter.
  - Record cycloplegic retinoscopic results for each eye.
  - Remove half of the retinoscopic working distance lenses (+0.75 D).
- Occlude OS and perform monocular manifest refraction (MMR) on OD.
  - After reaching the MMR endpoint for OD, occlude OD and perform MMR on OS.
- Record the cycloplegic MMR result and the corresponding distance visual acuity for each eye. (If cycloplegic results do not correspond with noncycloplegic results, rely more on the cycloplegic examination for refractive surgical data.)

KERATOMETRY

Indications
- necessary for calculations for intraocular lens implant for clear lens extraction.
- determination of the amount and location of corneal astigmatism
  - especially useful if a computerized corneal topographer is unavailable
  - comparison of the amount and location of corneal astigmatism with that of manifest refraction cylinder
- refractive astigmatism
- determination of central corneal power (steepness), which is especially useful for determining the type of microkeratome to use for laser in situ keratomileusis (LASIK)
- determining the integrity of the corneal/tear film surface
  - regular corneal surface and high quality tear film indicated by clear and regular corneal mires
  - an irregular corneal surface or poor tear film quality indicated by blurred irregular corneal mires (a possible *contraindication* to corneal refractive surgery)

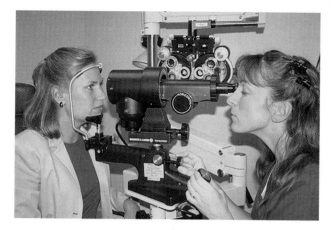

Figure 6–8 A patient being examined with a manual keratometer to diagnose the location, type, and amount of corneal cylinder. (Corneal mire quality can also be evaluated. It should be remembered that the keratometer only analyzes the central 3mm of the cornea.)

Methods (Fig. 6–8)

- Place the patient's head in the headrest of the keratometer.
- Instruct patient to look at their eye reflected at the end of the tube.
- With one of the patient's eyes occluded, focus the mires of the keratometer on the cornea of the unoccluded eye.
- Adjust the keratometer dials to achieve the correct alignment of the mires.
- Read the keratometry (K) values from the dials.

COMPUTERIZED CORNEAL TOPOGRAPHY

Indications

- far superior for most refractive surgical procedures because manual keratometry provides information about only the central 3 mm of the cornea
- determines the amount, location, regularity, and type of corneal astigmatism (Figs. 6–9 and 6–10)
- determination of central corneal power
  - helps select the best microkeratome for LASIK
  - helps determine pre- versus postoperative corneal changes

- helps screen out excessively flat corneas that may not be best treated with refractive procedures that primarily involve further corneal flattening
- screening out of preoperative corneal pathology
- identifies *forme fruste* keratoconus, which often appears as a steep (>47.00 D) inferior nasal apex with irregular astigmatism on corneal topography [a contraindication for refractive surgery especially photorefractive keratectomy (PRK) and LASIK] (Fig. 6–11)
  - identification of individuals with suspected keratoconus (more than 2.5 D of variation between the superior and inferior K values)
- evaluation of postoperative corneal condition
  - especially helps determine the presence or absence of central islands after excimer laser procedures, which are associated with residual myopia (Fig. 6–12)
  - helps determine the presence of a decentered ablation after laser refractive surgery (PRK or LASIK) (Fig. 6–13)
  - helps determine the presence of irregular corneal astigmatism following incisional keratotomy procedures, which may account for poor postoperative acuity

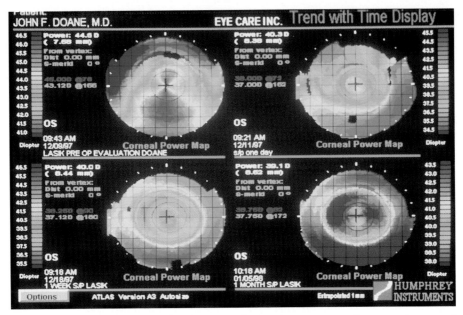

Figure 6–9 A computer topographical printout shows a large amount of preoperative corneal "within-the-rule" astigmatism and the trend-with-time topographical maps after LASIK.

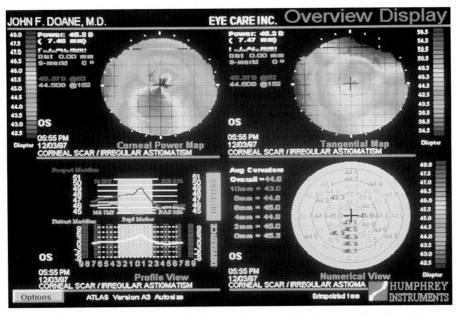

Figure 6–10 A computer topographical printout of a cornea showing irregular astigmatism secondary to a corneal scar.

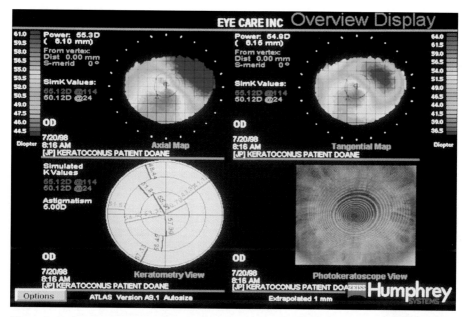

Figure 6–11 A computer topographical printout showing an inferior, steep nasal apex (>47.00 D). This patient has keratoconus.

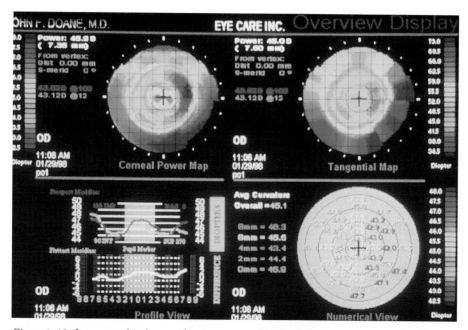

Figure 6–12 A topographical map of a cornea 3 weeks after LASIK that shows a steep central island. The patient showed residual myopia upon manifest refraction.

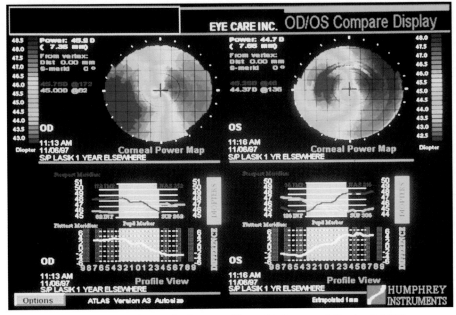

Figure 6–13 A topographical map of a decentered laser ablation zone following LASIK.

• evaluation of the integrity of the tear film/corneal surface interface
  ○ possible to view reflected corneal mires using the photokeratoscopic view available on most computerized corneal topographers (Fig. 6–14) [indication of a regular corneal surface (normal tear film clear and regular mires) and an irregular corneal surface (abnormal tear film blurred and irregular mires), which may adversely affect surgical results]
• individual assessment of the type and severity of corneal surface abnormalities

Methods
• Place the patient's head in the headrest.
• With one of the patient's eyes occluded, focus and center the reflected images on the cornea of the unoccluded eye.
• Capture and process the focused and centered image in the computer.

KERATOSCOPY

Indications
• identification of corneal mires using a battery-powered, light-emitting diode device (Maloney or Van Loenen keratoscopes; JEDMED Instrument Company, St. Louis, MO) that attaches to a standard slit lamp for a magnified, coaxial view or is hand held
• determination of corneal surface regularity and tear film quality for pre- and postoperative evaluations (corneal surface or tear film abnormalities indicated by irregular blurred mires a possible *contraindication* for some procedures because they suggest irregular astigmatism or keratoconus)

Methods
• Place the keratoscope in front of the eye to be tested.

REFRACTIVE SURGERY: A COLOR SYNOPSIS

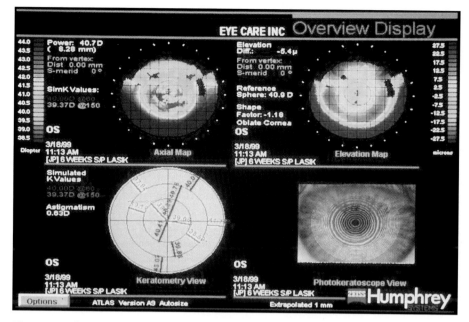

Figure 6–14 A computer printout of topographical analysis of a cornea that has poor quality tear film/surface interaction. Note the photokeratoscopic view (lower right) and the blurred, inconsistent mire circles reflected off the cornea.

- Adjust the distance of the keratoscope from the eye until the mires are focused.
- Note the configuration of the mires.

PACHYMETRY

Indications

- evaluation of corneal thickness (540 μm is normal), which guides or impacts some refractive surgery procedures (best to use solid-state ultrasonic pachymeters that are contact activated without a foot pedal, have a digital display, and have the ability to store and print out serial readings, e.g., pachymeters from Zeiss Humphrey Systems, Dublin, CA, or Sonogage, Cleveland, OH) (Fig. 6–15)
  - minimum values important for excimer laser refractive procedures (PRK and LASIK), especially in cases where intended ablation correction exceeds a spherical equivalent of 6.00 D
  - minimum to maximum (thinnest to thickest) values important for guiding incision depth and order of incisional keratotomy procedures [radial keratotomy (RK) and astigmatic keratotomy (AK); watch for variations of >75 μm; see Chapter 8]
  - maximum values important for guiding incision depth for limbal relaxing incisions and for guiding initial incision depth for insertion of corneal ring segments (Intacs; KeraVision, Freemont, CA)
  - identification of exceptionally low pachymetry values in a patient with high "against the rule" astigmatism (suspected keratoconus)

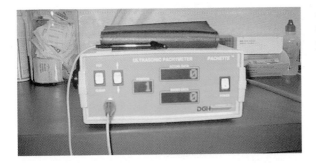

Figure 6–15 A solid-state, ultrasonic pachymeter with digital display and memory.

Methods
- Administer topical anesthesia (optional).
- Take multiple pachymetric readings to ensure consistency.
- Follow the manufacturer's suggested protocol for use and maintenance (Zeiss Humphrey Systems or Sonogage.)

SPECULAR MICROSCOPY

Indications
- documentation of endothelial cell count (normal range: at birth, 4,000–5,000 cells/mm^2; at 70–80 years, ~1000 cells/mm^2).
- identifies patients with decreased cell counts (i.e., severe gutatta or chronic contact lens wear) and, therefore, risk for developing corneal decompensation and bullous keratopathy (Fig. 6–16) (recommended although corneal refractive surgery is not known to significantly

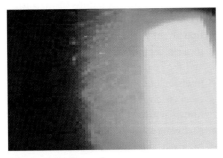

Figure 6–16 Corneal gutatta.

decrease endothelial cell counts more quickly than normal aging)
- identification of inadvertent trauma to the corneal endothelium during clear lens extraction (i.e., cataract surgery), which occasionally causes corneal decompensation and bullous keratopathy (severely depressed endothelial cell count is a *contraindication* for clear lens extraction as elective surgery)

ULTRASONIC SCANNING

A-Scans
Indications
- quantification of the axial length of the eye [normal axial length: 21 to 26 mm; <20 mm indicates a *nanophthalmic* (short) eye; >26.5 mm indicates a *macrophthalmic* (long) eye]
  - <0.3 mm difference between eyes (1.0 mm of difference equals ~3.0 D of difference in eyeglass prescription for each eye)
  - diagnosis of axial anisometropia by comparing the axial length of the OU
- critical accurate measurement of nanophthalmic eyes because power of the IOL increases inversely with axial length
- difficult measurement of longest part of a macrophthalmic eye (usually not at the fovea because the eye tends to bulge posteriorly and temporally forming a staphyloma; important length is the distance between the corneal apex and fovea)

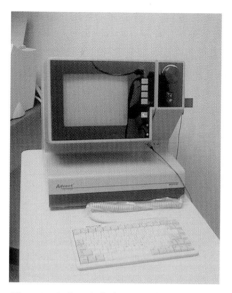

Figure 6–17 A typical ultrasound A/B-scan unit.

• quantification of the depth of the anterior chamber, and thickness of the lens by most units (e.g., DGH 500 A-Scan; DGH Technology, Inc., Exton, PA) (Fig. 6–17)
• necessary for IOL implant calculations in clear lens extraction

APPLANATION A-SCANS

Indications

• required for measurement of the front surface of the cornea (Fig. 6–18)
• minimization of risk for obtaining artificially short axial length measurements because of corneal indentation during applanation of the corneal surface by using an available spring-loaded mount on the probe

IMMERSION A-SCANS

Indications

• generally better accuracy because of lack of corneal indentation but slightly more complicated to operate than an applanation A-scan because of the need of creating an immersion waterbath over the eye
• possibility of poor echo readings with extra fluid around the eye because the ultrasound waves must travel through more dense media to get to the eye

Methods

• Place a water bath around the eye to avoid direct corneal indentation (Fig. 6–19).
• Take multiple measurements to ensure consistancy.

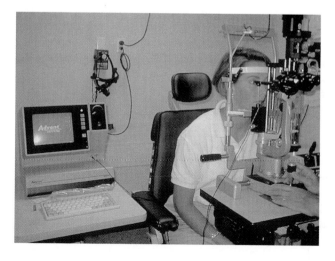

Figure 6–18 An applanation A-scan technique being performed on a patient with mounted probe.

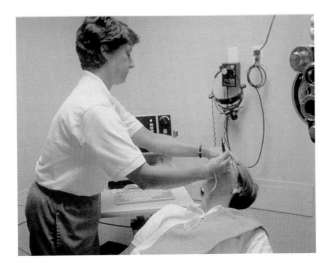

Figure 6–19 Immersion A-scan technique being performed on a patient by a technician.

B-Scans

Indications

- best for acquisition of axial length data for highly myopic surgical candidates who have macrophthalmic eyes because of posterior staphyloma and the possibility of inaccurate A-scan data
- availability of A-scan capabilities with many late model B-scan units (see Fig. 6–17)

Methods

- Put an electronic mark on the apex of the cornea (possible with most B-scan units).
- For eyes with an axial length of more than 26.5 mm, measure 4.5 mm temporally from the center of the optic nerve and place another electronic mark at that point on the retina for each eye (the center of the optic nerve and the fovea are about 4.5 mm apart).
- The difference between the two electronic marks is the "true" axial length of the eye, the distance between the fovea and the corneal apex instead of the distance between the posterior portion of the staphyloma and the corneal apex.
- Repeat for the other eye.

HIGH-FREQUENCY ANTERIOR SEGMENT ULTRASOUND BIOMICROSCOPY

Indications

- determination of the exact anatomical relationship among the posterior iris and anterior lens capsule, anterior chamber depth, and anterior chamber angle anatomy
- preoperative evaluation for implantation of an intraocular contact lens (ICL) behind the iris and in front of the natural lens to correct myopic or hyperopic refractive error while still allowing for accommodation (STAAR Surgical Co., Monrovia, CA; currently undergoing investigative trials)

Methods

- Cover the closed anesthetized eye with ultrasound gel supplied by the manufacturer of the probe.
- Place the ultrasonic probe over the closed, anesthetized eye.
- Maintain the appropriate angulation of the probe (90 degrees to the surface being examined), which will yield the sharpest image.

CONTRAST SENSITIVITY TESTING

Indications

• evaluation of a patient's visual function for different levels of contrast
  ○ incorporation of sinusoidal gratings that proceed from low spatial frequency to high spatial frequency going down the chart vertically (most charts)
  ○ variation of contrast of the sinusoidal gratings from high to low, going left to right horizontally across the chart for each spatial frequency (most charts)
  ○ allows examiner to decide if prescription eyeglasses will help the patient's visual function under certain conditions (e.g., improved driving at night if contrast sensitivity is better with eyeglasses).
• commercial availability of many different types of contrast sensitivity charts and testing devices [some designed for near, some for distance, and some for both distance and near; some charts with illuminated backgrounds and remote-control devices, and others mounted on cardboard (Fig. 6–20)].
• especially valuable to evaluate impact of eyeglasses on vision if early cataracts or glaucoma are present
• evaluation of postoperative patients who complain of decreased vision in dimly lit conditions

Methods

• Follow the manufacturer's suggested instructions for use and grading (provided with test).
• Perform distance contrast sensitivity testing 10 feet from the chart.

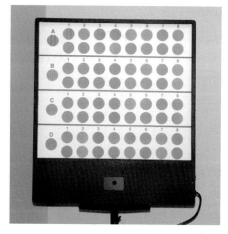

Figure 6–20 A remote-controlled contrast sensitivity chart with background illumination.

• Perform near testing usually 18 inches from the chart.
• Perform contrast sensitivity testing near and at distance with and without correction; in dim and bright lighting.

Suggested Readings

Assil KK, Schanzlin DJ. *Radial and Astigmatic Keratotomy: A Complete Handbook.* St. Louis, MO: Poole Press; 1994.

Carlson NS, Kurtz D, Heath DA, Hines C. *Clinical Procedures for Ocular Examination.* Norwalk, CT: Appleton & Lange; 1990.

Holladay JT. Why the A-scan is your key to better cataract care. *Rev Optometry.* 1999; 30:85–88.

Machat JJ, Slade SG, Probst LE. *The Art of LASIK.* 2nd ed. Thorofare, NJ: Slack Inc.; 1999.

CHAPTER 7

Operative Refraction Targets

Scot Morris, John F. Doane, Andrea D. Border, and James A. Denning

CHAPTER CONTENTS

Age Concerns

Selection of a Target

Multifocal Lenses

Suggested Readings

A thorough patient history is key to the success of refractive surgery. Preoperative patient assessment should include obtaining a complete ocular and systemic medical history as well as the patient's reasons for pursuing surgery and his or her postoperative expectations. Many surgical options are available (Table 7–1). This chapter discusses presbyopic considerations and how to determine the refractive target.

AGE CONCERNS

The chronological age of the patient's eye is a primary factor in the determination of

TABLE 7–1
Surgical Categories and Techniques.

Surgical Category	Techniques
Lamellar	Keratomileusis
	LASIK
	Intracorneal rings/segments
	Keratophakia
	Epikeratoplasty
	Lamellar keratoplasty
Incisional	Radial keratotomy
	Astigmatic keratotomy
	Limbal relaxation incisions
Keratectomy	Photorefractive keratectomy
Thermal keratoplasty	Holmium thermokeratoplasty
Intraocular implantation	Phakic intraocular lenses
	Refractive lensectomy

refractive target. Patients need to understand before surgery that age has a direct impact on the postoperative healing process. This is crucial to prevent unrealistic expectations.

Adolescence

Refractive procedures are not recommended for prepubertal and pubescent teenagers. Currently, some surgeons are evaluating refractive surgery for adolescents with strabismus, but it is too early to generally recommend this option.

Preoperative Considerations
- general ocular health
- progression of refractive error
- refractive stability
- visual demands and working distances
- accommodation
- need for extreme caution with patients in late adolescence (refraction often unstable)

Adulthood

Refractive targets for adults vary widely from full-distance correction for young adults to monovision considerations with presbyopic patients.

PREPRESBYOPIC ADULTS Prepresbyopic adults are usually 20 to 40 years of age.

Preoperative Considerations
- patient education about the effects and progression of presbyopia and mechanisms of correction (reading glasses, monovision with contact lenses, surgically induced monovision, multifocal options)
- refractive stability
- progression of refractive error secondary to high demand for near tasks
- occupational and recreational visual demands (e.g., sufficiency of accommodation for near tasks, need for binocularity)
- speed of progressive loss of accommodation from hyperopia (in patient's mid 30s)

to emmetropia (in patient's early 40s) to myopia (in patient's mid to late 40s)
- ocular health (early cataracts, trauma, or ocular surface disease)

PRESBYOPIC ADULTS Presbyopia usually begins to affect adults in their early to mid 40s.

Preoperative Considerations
- refractive stability (more stable unless active ocular disease is present)
- speed and progressive nature of loss of accommodation
- absolute presbyopia by age 65
- patient education about the effects and progression of presbyopia and mechanisms of correction (reading glasses, monovision with contact lenses, surgically induced monovision, multifocal options)
- patient education (about need for reading glasses if bilateral distance refraction is the target)
- patient willingness to sacrifice bilateral acute distance vision for functional vision without correction at multiple distances
- adaptability to monovision
- increased frequency of ocular diseases in older age groups, including cataracts and age-related macular degeneration

SELECTION OF A TARGET

Determination of the refractive target may be the most important part of the presurgical patient examination. Discussion of various target options follows.

Bilateral Distance Target
The bilateral distance target is the most common option for full-distance correction and elimination of all refractive error in both eyes.

Preoperative Considerations

- ocular dominance (less critical because both eyes are corrected for distance)
- desire for optimal binocular distance vision (the reason most young adults and many presbyopic adults choose surgery)
- visual recreational and occupational demands (especially important in prepresbyopic and presbyopic individuals)
- evaluation of binocular status to rule out binocular abnormality and avoid patient expectation of no longer needing to wear eyeglasses
- possibility of diplopia in some patients with anisometropia and compensatory suppression in those with mild to moderate phorias or an alternating tropia (may require full-time prismatic correction postoperatively)
- documentation of possible postoperative effects on binocular vision if binocular abnormality found at preoperative assessment
- patient education about the advantages and disadvantages of binocular distance vision to prevent the surprise of decreased postoperative near visual acuity
- demonstration of patient's postoperative vision with trial frames or contact lenses to show the effect of distance correction on near vision
- addition of a 1- to 1.5-D myopic lens in both eyes to simulate loss of accommodative reserve, especially for prepresbyopic patients

Bilateral Near or Intermediate Target

Though less frequently pursued, some individuals choose to have bilateral near or intermediate targets. Bilateral near or intermediate vision may be useful for certain occupations that require prolonged near-vision tasks (e.g., a computer programmer or professional pianist).

Preoperative Considerations

- demonstration of less than optimal distance vision using trial frames or contact lenses to create proper patient expectations
- patient education about the need for distance prescription eyeglasses or part-time contact lens wear to maximize distance acuity for driving and other distance tasks (verbal acknowledgment by the patient and chart documentation are essential)

Monovision

For decades contact lens wearers have utilized monovision to achieve functional vision at variable distances.

Preoperative Considerations

- ocular dominance (dominant eye usually corrected for distance and nondominant eye corrected for near and/or intermediate distance, although some may prefer dominant eye for near if majority of time spent doing near tasks)
- extensive patient education about advantages and disadvantages of monovision and proper candidate selection
- preoperative trial and acceptance of postoperative vision using contact lenses or trial eyeglasses (Fig. 7–1)
- patient tolerance of mild distance blur, photopic blur/night myopia, and progression of presbyopia
- patient's reason for pursuing surgery (ideal candidate: desire to be rid of eyeglasses completely or to minimize or forestall their use for near-visual tasks and a lack of hypercritical concern about visual requirements; poor candidate: need for excellent depth perception or acute vision at certain distances)
- ability to accept a sacrifice in binocularity and resolution at all distances because of induced mild anisometropia (varies considerably among individuals)

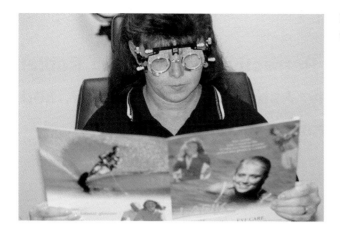

Figure 7–1 Monovision trial with trial frames.

MULTIFOCAL LENSES

Although not currently the standard method of refractive surgery, the use of intraocular multifocal lenses also warrants discussion.

Advantages
- marked decrease in need for any form of additional optical correction
- potential for inducing mild blur at all distances and glare from the transi-tional component of the intraocular lens (IOL)
- extensive interest in the refractive community in multifocal IOLs with cataract extraction and clear lens extraction

Disadvantages
- requirement of extensive education to educate patients about potential complications with these lenses
  - loss of best corrected acuity
  - loss of contrast sensitivity
  - disabling night glare

Suggested Readings

Demers PE, Wu HK, Steinert RF. Refractive error. In: Wu HK, Thompson VM, Steinert RF, Slade SD, Hersh PS, eds. *Refractive Surgery.* New York: Thieme; 1999:3–39.

CHAPTER 8

Incisional Refractive Techniques: Radial Keratotomy, Astigmatic Keratotomy, and Limbal Relaxing Incisions

Kerry K. Assill, Andrea D. Border, John F. Doane, Scot Morris, and James A. Denning

CHAPTER CONTENTS

Radial keratotomy (RK) and astigmatic keratotomy (AK) were the first refractive procedures to be practiced on a wide scale in North America. Although photorefractive RK and laser in situ keratomileusis have largely replaced these two procedures, they are still effective for low myopia and astigmatism and are occasionally used by refractive surgeons. Most of the concepts now used for refractive surgery were developed originally for RK and AK.

GENERAL PREOPERATIVE CONSIDERATIONS

Indications
• low to moderate myopia and/or astigmatism
• realistic patient expectations of surgical effect
• patient age greater than 21 years

Patient Evaluation
• documented medical history (see list of contraindications on pages 69–70)
• family history (especially of keratoconus or rheumatoid arthritis)
• measurement of distance and near uncorrected visual acuity (for statistical documentation, postoperative patient comparison, and legal considerations)
• manifest refraction and, ideally, cycloplegic refraction [after discontinuation of rigid gas-permeable (RGP) contact lens wear for 3 weeks and soft contact lens (SCL) wear for 3 days]
• evaluate for potential problems using corneal topography (e.g., keratoconus, irregular astigmatism, and contact lens warpage)
  ○ Retest every 2 to 3 weeks until stable using corneal topography, after discontinuing contact lens wear (also

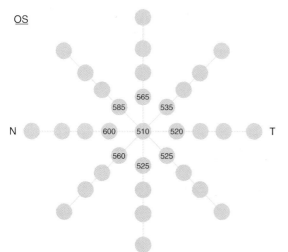

OS

N

T

Figure 8–1 The eight paracentral meridia viewed serially by pachymetry from superotemporal to superior.

helps determine the meridian and zone for arcuate and tangential incisions)

- slit-lamp examination (rules out any pre-existing corneal disease)
- dilated fundus examination (rules out any macular or peripheral retinal disease)
- serial pachymetry at the corneal apex and at eight paracentral meridia (from superotemporal to superior) to determine the thinnest paracentral zone [Be alert for serial readings differing more than 75 μm (Fig. 8–1).]
- tonometry [establishes preoperative baseline intraocular pressure (IOP); increased IOP may result in greater than expected refractive results]
- determination of ocular dominance (see Chapter 5)
- patient education
  - one-on-one conferences
  - educational brochures
  - videos
  - ample opportunity for patient questions (and answers from knowledgeable personnel)
- informed consent read by patient in its entirety and signed in ink; personally reviewed by surgeon with the patient and signed in the patient's presence by surgeon

Patient Preparation
- Administer broad-spectrum antibiotics for prophylaxis approximately 25 minutes before surgery.
- Instill 1% pilocarpine.
  - ensures maximum patient focus intraoperatively with high illumination
  - better defines patient's visual axis
- Apply topical anesthetic but not directly to the corneal epithelium [recommended regime: 1 gtt of 4% lidocaine (Xylocaine; Abbott) every 10 minutes (×2), followed by 1 gtt of 0.5% tetracaine every 10 minutes (×2)].
- Administer up to 20 mg of diazepam 20 minutes before surgery (acts as an anxiolytic and relaxes the muscles of the eye to make the lid speculum more comfortable).

GENERAL SURGICAL CONSIDERATIONS

Relative Contraindications
- tendency toward aggressive wound healing due to potential minimized effect and a greater potential for future hyperopic drift

- collagen vascular disease [propensity for stromal melt (keratolysis) following the procedure]
- active infectious or inflammatory ocular conditions (e.g., blepharoconjunctivitis or ocular rosacea, which should be fully controlled before surgery)

Absolute Contraindications
- unrealistic patient expectations of perfect vision or improved best corrected visual acuity (BCVA)
- patient age less than 21 years
- systemic disease (e.g., diabetes mellitus because of possible poor healing of corneal incisions)
- recent unstable refraction greater than 0.5 D sphere or cylinder (within the previous 24 months)
- keratoconus because of progressive ectasia
- corneal warpage from contact lens wear or large, chronic eyelid masses like chalazia (discontinue lens wear and topographically document stable curvature before surgery)
- preexisting irregular astigmatism
- severe retinopathy
  ○ increased risk for severely compromised acuity in the future
  ○ possible adverse effects on low contrast acuity from increased depth of focus
- severe dry eye (keratoconjunctivitis sicca)
  ○ increased risk for keratolysis
  ○ greatly prolonged visual recovery
- history of chronic herpes simplex or zoster keratitis because of the increased risk for keratolysis (ideally should not be considered for surgery)

Equipment
- a user-friendly computerized topographer
- an operating microscope (with certain features)
  ○ a para-axial illumination source

○ an infrared filter (prevents corneal desiccation)
○ an ultraviolet filter (eliminates retinal phototoxicity)
○ a coaxial fixation target
- durable optical zone (OZ) and radial markers machined from a single sheet of titanium (without soldered cross hairs or gold plating)
- a corneal pachymeter (with certain features)
  ○ a solid-state probe
  ○ continuous readout
  ○ contact activation
  ○ a display monitor
  ○ enough memory for multiple readings
- a combined-style diamond knife (with certain features)
  ○ a 45-degree-angle head
  ○ 80 to 120 μm thick
  ○ retractable for safe handling
  ○ universal design footplates
  ○ a high quality diamond blade (Fig. 8–2)
- a computer-programmable diamond knife with computer-driven motor (allows the pachymeter to communicate with the diamond to reduce microperforations and improve topographic profiles; now superceded by the excimer laser)

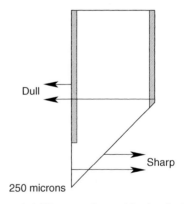

Figure 8–2 Diagram of a combined-style diamond knife.

Methods

- Position the patient comfortably on the operating table with a folded towel or foam pillow under the neck to facilitate the chin-up position required for placement of superior incisions.
- Patch the nonsurgical eye.
- A trained, gloved, and masked technician may administer periocular povidone iodine solution (Betadine).
- Wipe away excess solution.
- Position the open, sterile eye drape over the patient's face.
- Immediately before beginning the actual procedure, instill 1 final drop of 0.5% tetracaine into the conjunctiva.
- Position a lid speculum to allow adequate ocular exposure and avoid undue eyelid tension.
- Use one of the three methods that follow to mark the exact center of the pupil (i.e., the visual axis).
- Use the miotic pupil centering method.
  - Instill a miotic agent, such as 1% pilocarpine.
  - Mark the exact center of the pupil (miotic pupil centering).
- Use the light filament reflex method (recommended by the PERK Study Group).
  - Physically mark the midpoint along the lower margin of the reflex on the cornea while the patient fixates on the microscope light filament.
  - Look through one ocular and mark along the opposite inferior border of the light filament reflex [e.g., if you fixate through the left ocular, the mark should be positioned along the lower right border of the filament reflex on the cornea (Fig. 8–3)].
- Use the coaxial light source method.
  - This method allows the patient to fixate on a less intense light during the procedure than does the light filament reflex method and is more precise.

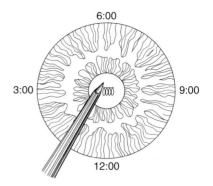

Figure 8–3 When looking through the left ocular, the surgeon marks the visual axis along the opposite inferior border of the filament reflex on the cornea.

  - Coaxially mount a fixation light source between the patient and the surgeon within the operating microscope optical system.
- Mark the visual axis as follows.
  - When the lid speculum is in place, administer 1 drop of balanced salt solution (BSS) over the corneal apex to enhance the corneal light reflex.
  - Use a Sinskey hook to carefully indent the epithelium overlying the visual axis.
  - Mark the axis carefully because any deep epithelial defect can leave scarring in the visual axis.
  - When the epithelial indentation is not easily visible, use a Weck cell sponge to dry the central epithelium and enhance visualization.
  - Clear excess pooling in the canthal region with a Weck cell sponge (a dry field is important for detection of early microperforation).
  - Avoid excessive dryness to decrease friction between knife footplates and corneal epithelium.
- Identify and mark the OZ.
  - Align the cross hairs of the OZ marker with the visual axis epithelial marking.

- Apply proper pressure to the OZ marker to avoid misalignment. (Misalignment commonly occurs when the visual axis does not coincide with the corneal apex and when slippage occurs across the epithelium because of improper pressure.)
- Use a Weck cell sponge to gently dry the epithelium and enhance markings (as with all pressure-induced markings, moisture may cause the indentations to become faint).
- Ensure proper globe centration (improper centration contributes to decentration of the OZ marking).
- Perform corneal pachymetry.
  - Soak the probe tip in hydrogen peroxide.
  - Dry the tip with an alcohol wipe.
  - Allow the tip to air dry.
  - Position the probe tip exactly perpendicular to the epithelium at 1.5 mm temporal to the visual axis and at the thinnest paracentral point (determined by preoperative pachymetery screening).
  - If pachymetry readings do not register, ensure that the probe tip is *exactly* perpendicular with the corneal epithelium or moisten the epithelium with a microdrop of BSS.
  - Usually the thinnest paracentral site corresponds with the paracentral temporal site, but if these two sites differ in thickness, set the diamond blade to 100% of the thinner of the two (use a calibrating microscope to set the blade).
  - When the range of paracentral screening values (from thickest to thinnest) is greater than 75 μm, expect less refractive change than predicted by the nomogram, and lengthen the incisions slightly toward the limbus or reduce the recommended optical zone by 0.25 mm.
- Calibrate and adjust the diamond knife.
  - Sterilize and mount the diamond knife into the sterile mounting block of the calibrating microscope at the beginning of each procedure.
  - Zero the knife footplates and either extend the diamond to 550 μm or set it to correspond with the thinnest paracentral screening pachymetery reading.
  - After obtaining real-time intraoperative pachymetry readings, adjust the diamond tip accordingly.
  - Make the final setting of the diamond knife blade 100% of the thinnest *intraoperative* pachymetery reading.
- If consistent undercorrections result but without microperforations or incisions approaching the pre-Descemet's region, set the diamond blade to a longer setting (in 10-μm or 2% increments) for subsequent incisional procedures on other patients.
  - If consistent undercorrections occur with deep incisions or incisions that extend within 1 mm of the limbus, decrease the OZ diameter by 0.25 mm.

GENERAL POSTOPERATIVE CONSIDERATIONS

Medications
- 1 drop neomycin/poly/dexamethasone (Maxitrol); 1 drop diclofenac sodium (Voltaren; Cibavison), 1 drop aminoglycoside, or 1 drop fluoroquinolone
- 1 drop Voltaren every 6 hours as needed for pain (first evening only)
- 1 drop Maxitrol every 6 hours for 5 days and then every 12 hours for 2 days only (same schedule for aminoglycoside or fluoroquinolone, which may be taken several minutes after Maxitrol)
- 2 oxycodone/acetaminophen (Percocet) tabs every 6 hours for immediate postoperative pain (optional)

Patient Instructions

- Provide written instructions to the patient.
- Instruct patient to go home and sleep for several hours and to take the drops as directed (see above).
- Instruct patient not to rub his or her eyes.
- Instruct patient not to use eye make-up for 2 weeks.
- Instruct patient to avoid contaminated water (e.g., pools, hot tubs, showers) for 2 weeks.
- Instruct patient to refrain from reading for the first day after surgery.
- Instruct patient to call emergency telephone numbers if experiencing severe pain, discharge, increased redness, or swelling.
- Inform patient about first follow-up visit.

Follow-Up

- first postoperative visit (day 2)
  - Measure uncorrected acuity.
  - Perform a slit-lamp examination.
- subsequent postoperative visits (weeks 1, 3, and 6 and months 3, 6, and 12)
  - Schedule for late afternoon for corneal stability.
  - Measure uncorrected visual acuity.
  - Measure manifest refraction.
  - Measure BCVA.
  - Perform slit-lamp examination.
  - Review patient progress and symptoms.

Enhancements

- nonsurgical
  - Nonsurgical intervention is possible if the degree of myopia is within 0.5 D of target.
  - Begin with pressure patching (preferred) beginning at 1 week and continuing for 6 weeks only at night or continuously both day and night.
- surgical
  - Surgery is required if residual myopia is greater than 0.5 D.

- Provide additional incisions (cumulative total, ≤ 8) if the undercorrection is greater than 1.25 D, the OZ is a minimum of 2.75 mm, the limbal zone is a minimum of 0.5 mm, and there are fewer than eight original incisions.
- Lengthen existing incisions by decreasing the limbal clear zone or by decreasing the optical clear zone (if the undercorrection is 0.50–1.25 D, the OZ is >2.75 mm, the limbal zone is >0.5 mm, and there is significant astigmatism and eight original incisions).
- Deepen some or all of the existing incisions if they appear to be shallow at the slit lamp, the OZ is at the minimum, and there are at least eight original incisions.

RADIAL KERATOTOMY

Preoperative Considerations
Indications
- particularly effective for up to -4 D of myopia
- increasingly effective with increasing age
- best to aim for slight undercorrection to compensate for the progressive hyperopic shift documented with RK (0.1 D/year)

Surgical Considerations
Methods
- Center radial markings to the optical zone marker (based on the nomogram) and place in contact with the corneal epithelium with moderate pressure for several seconds.
- Perform radial incisions.
  - Because the cornea thins progressively during the procedure, incise the thinnest corneal quadrant first and the thickest quadrant last (thinnest to thickest) to minimize perforation risk.
  - For an ideal incision, terminate the incision 1 mm inside the limbus at a constant depth within 85% to 90% of

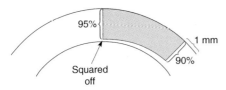

Figure 8–4 Diagram of the base of a radial incision being squared off.

stromal depth throughout the length of the cut.

- ○ The central extent of the incision should slightly undermine the OZ.
- ○ Square off the base of the incision and extend it centrally beyond the surface OZ margin (Fig. 8–4).
- ○ Achieving ideal incision characteristics minimizes the risks of fibrovascular ingrowth into incisions and undercorrections.
- Use the combined (genesis) technique.
- ○ The centripetal (Russian) incision begins at the limbus and progresses toward the OZ [provides reliably deeper incisions than does the centrifugal (American) incision (Fig. 8–5)].
- ○ The centrifugal (American) incision begins at the optical zone and progresses toward the limbus [safer than the Russian incision because it rarely invades the central clear zone (Fig. 8–6)].
- ○ The diamond knife design for this combined technique allows for both centripetal and centrifugal incisions to be performed with the same blade because of its vector force–sensitive design. The knife cuts along the entire centrifugal (angled) margin and along the distal 250 μm of the centripetal (vertical) margin (see Fig. 8–2).
- ○ First perform the centrifugal incision, beginning at the optical zone and ending 1 mm inside the limbus (Fig. 8–7A) (results in an inconsistently deep but relatively shallow "safety" groove of

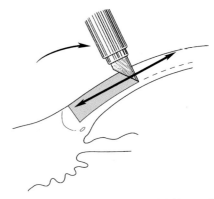

Figure 8–5 Diagram of a centripetal (Russian) incision.

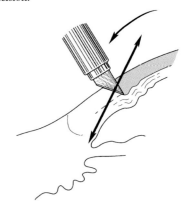

Figure 8–6 Diagram of a centrifugal (American) incision.

inconsistent depth that helps to guide the centripetal incision.).

- ○ At the termination of the first (centrifugal) incision, keep the blade in the groove.
- ○ Reverse the motion to begin the centripetal incision toward the optical zone. [This second incision deepens and evens out the groove (Fig. 8–7B). During the second incision, it is nearly impossible to veer outside of the first groove or to incise beyond the initiation of the first incision into the optical zone. The uphill centripetal incision also ensures uniform depth and a slight undermining of the optical zone for maximal effect (Fig. 8–7C).]

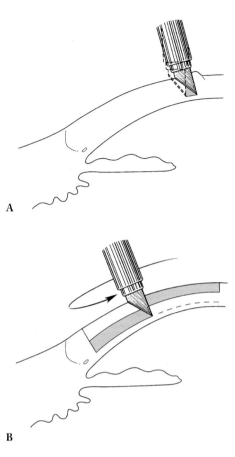

A

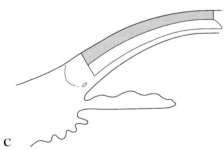

B

C

Figure 8–7 A combined (genesis) incision. (A) The centrifugal incision begins at the OZ. (B) Keeping the blade in the groove, the second incision deepens and evens out the groove. (C) The uphill centripetal incision ensures uniform depth and slight undermining of the OZ for maximal effect.

- Use the ideal combined technique.
  - Insert the combined-style diamond blade (tip points posterocentrally) at the OZ margin slightly oblique to the corneal surface.
  - Apply pressure while penetrating posterocentrally and pause for 1 second.
  - Gently undermine the OZ.
  - Reorient the diamond blade perpendicular to the corneal epithelium.
  - Initiate the centrifugal incision directed toward the limbus.
  - Terminate the centrifugal incision 1 mm short of the limbus.
  - Return toward the OZ with centripetal motion within the groove.
  - Gently undermine the OZ again.
  - Remove the diamond blade from the groove by pulling away from OZ.
- Control microtremors.
  - Use both hands on diamond knife (when using guarded diamond for RK).
  - Use a wrist rest.
  - Rest hands on the patient's face.
  - Relax your shoulders and exhale slowly.
  - Use a mild Valsalva maneuver.
  - Unless contraindicated, self-administer beta blocker drops 10 minutes before the procedure.

Intraoperative Complications

- invasion of incisions into the optical zone (caused by inaccurate visual axis marking or spontaneous patient eye movement and may lead to several postoperative complications); to avoid, ensure proper globe centration when marking visual axis and avoid parallax errors and use the combined (genesis) technique (see pages 74–75) to minimize risk for eye movement.
  - increased glare
  - irregular astigmatism
  - monocular diplopia (possible)
- incisions extending into the limbus (caused by incising beyond clear cornea)

- corneal destabilization over time from fibrovascular ingrowth
- large diurnal fluctuations
- progression of effect
- intersecting incisions
  - wound gape
  - poor healing
  - If either occurs, reapproximate the wound edges with 10-0 or 11-0 nylon sutures left in place for 10 to 12 weeks.
- corneal perforation (more easily recognized in a relatively dry field)
  - Microperforations self seal and do not show a leak on a dry Weck cell. (Treat with cycloplegia, use topical aqueous suppressants and antibiotics, and cover with a fox shield.
  - Larger perforations leak on Weck cell challenge and require suture closure, antibiotics, cycloplegia, and coverage with a fox shield.
- diamond blade chipping [rare but possibly caused by a blade that is too thin or has been mishandled (e.g., scraped against metal)]
- optic nerve damage (especially in highly myopic eyes and associated with retrobulbar anesthesia, which is *not* indicated for use in performing incisional keratotomy)

Postoperative Considerations
Complications
- prevention
  - Do not cross incisions.
  - Do not incise to limbus.
  - Do not redeepen periphery.
  - Do not ignore microperforation.
  - Do not operate on a wet field.
- adhere to sterile techniques, instill prophylactic antibiotics on the day of surgery, instruct patients to avoid potentially infective water for 2 weeks postoperatively, avoid chronic topical steroids, and discourage postoperative contact lens wear (for infectious keratitis)

- self-limited complications
  - halo/starbursting (to minimize, stage the procedure with variable incisions and use a larger OZ; possibly caused by irregular astigmatism)
  - diurnal visual fluctuation (usually occurs in the first weeks to months but may be permanent) and is caused by immature wound architecture and variable corneal edema but diminishes as wounds mature; older patients may be hyperopic in the morning; encourage patients not to rub their eyes)
  - early regression (characterized by better vision in the morning and increased myopia toward evening; overcorrected older patients are hyperopic with symptoms throughout the day, whereas younger patients are more symptomatic in the morning; patients should avoid rubbing their eyes)
- non–sight threatening complications
  - undercorrection (usually requires enhancement)
  - overcorrection (may be controlled with epinephrine or propine 4 times a day for 6 weeks to simulate myofibroblast contraction and with 0.5%–1% pilocarpine 4 times a day to lower IOP, which may accelerate the regression of effect; may be necessary to open and scrape out fibrous tissue from within the groove and reapproximate margins with suture closure)
  - regression of effect (caused by early wound closure; operate on the patient's nondominant eye first and adjust the technique accordingly for the patient's dominant eye)
  - progression of effect (less common because incisions often do not extend into the limbus; treat by reopening wounds, removing fibrovascular tissue, and resuturing the wound; patients should avoid contact lens wear before and after surgery)

- regular or irregular induced astigmatism (usually self-limiting but risk increases with fewer incisions, a decentered OZ, or irregular incisions, long incisions, and crossed incisions
- miscellaneous other complications
  - contact lens intolerance
  - epithelial basement membrane dystrophy
  - epithelial inclusion cysts
  - foreign particles within grooves
  - epithelial iron lines
  - diminished corneal strength
  - endothelial cell loss
- sight-threatening complications
  - keratolysis [often occurs among patients with crossed incisions but also found among patients with rheumatoid arthritis or other collagen vascular diseases associated with keratoconjunctivitis sicca (these patients not considered as good candidates)]
  - infectious keratitis (treat aggressively with culture and sensitivity of the stromal infiltrates and frequent broad-spectrum topical antibiotics)

Enhancements
- Perform no more than two enhancements per eye.
- Make no more than a total of eight incisions (primary plus enhancements).
- The limbal zone must be a minimum of 0.5 mm.
- The OZ must be a minimum 2.75 mm.

ASTIGMATIC KERATOTOMY

Preoperative Considerations
Preoperative care for AK is identical to that for RK patients.

Indications
- myopic or plano-spherical equivalent refraction

- astigmatic patients intolerant of contact lenses (high cylinder in the spectacle plane creates peripheral vision problems)

Patient Preparation
- Determine the axis of astigmatism using corneal topography, manifest refraction, and cycloplegic refractive results.
- Perform a case-by-case analysis if these three methods reveal disparate axes.
- For orthogonal astigmatism, use manifest refraction cylinder axis.
- For nonorthogonal astigmatism (two steep hemimeridia differ by >180 degrees), use the topographical map cylinder if consistent with refraction in its sphero-cylindrical reconstruction.
- Rely on cycloplegic refractive cylinder to support use of manifest or topographical cylinder.
- Translate the determined axis to cornea.
  - Because the axis is determined with the patient upright and without sedation or a lid speculum, mark the cornea for axis with the patient in these same conditions to avoid serious axis positioning errors.
  - With the contralateral eye patched and the patient seated at a slit lamp, instill the anesthetic.
  - Adjust the slit-lamp light filament coaxial with the patient's eye.
  - To minimize accommodation, instruct the patient to fixate through the light filament at a distance.
  - Align the slit-lamp beam (vertically or horizontally) with the light filament.
- Carefully abrade the epithelium at the outer margins of the long axis of the beam using jeweler's forceps or a Sinskey hook. (In the operating room, this epithelial abrasion serves as the markings for the true 90-degree or 180-degree reference axis.)
- With the *true* axis in place, mark the predetermined actual astigmatism axis on the cornea (using an axis marker and surgical marking pen).

- To place arcuate incisions on patients with orthogonal astigmatism, use OZ radial markers to guide incision placement. (Use a four-wing marker for incisions at 90 degrees, a six-wing marker for 60 degrees, and an eight-wing marker for 45 degrees.)
- For patients with nonorthogonal astigmatism, mark the precise position to be incised with a degree-gauge marker and marking pen.
- Once markings are in place, perform pachymetry at the selected optical zone over the incision sites, and set the diamond blade at 100% of the thinner measurements.

Surgical Considerations
Methods
- Fixate the globe with two-point forceps grasping the conjunctiva near the limbus.
- Incise over the corneal marks with the diamond blade perpendicular to corneal stroma.
  - Achieve maximal effect with 5- to 7-mm OZs.
  - A 3-mm tangential incision yields the same effect as a 45-degree arcuate incision at a 6-mm optical zone.
  - Longer incisions and arcuate incisions are more efficient.
  - Longer incisions yield greater effect up to a 90-degree arc length.
  - AK incisions peripheral to old scars are ineffective.

Postoperative Considerations
Age and wound healing properties affect outcomes. For example, a 30-year-old patient should theoretically be compensated for effect: EFFECT = 100% + (patient age − 30) × 2%. Because the standard distribution of effect of AK is greater than that of RK, attempt only 60% of the full correction.

Postoperative Care
- Postoperative pharmacological care for AK patients is identical to that for RK patients (see page 72).
- Consider enhancements when applicable.

Enhancements
- Wait at least 6 weeks before attempting enhancements because AK enhancements require more time to stabilize than do radial incisions.
- Dilate patients because you will be able to more easily discern the incisions against a red reflex and avoid intersecting previous incisions.
- If postoperative topography maps show persistent irregular astigmatism in the original hemimeridian, a too-shallow or shelved incision is likely present. Properly place an adjacent incision in the same hemimeridian to correct this (possibly).
- If postoperative topography maps show a shift in astigmatism axis, irregular astigmatism, or undercorrection, use the topographical map to elongate the original incisions in the direction of the resultant steep zone.
- If the resultant refractive error is hyperopic astigmatism, cautiously reopen the original incisions , remove the fibrous plug, and reapproximate the wound margins using 10-0 nylon suture.
- Also, reapproximate wound margins using 10-0 nylon sutures (if the flat axis was incorrectly incised) unless the resultant refractive error is still myopic astigmatism. If so, place conservatively short arcuate incisions at the newly defined steep hemimeridia.

LIMBAL RELAXING INCISIONS

Preoperative Considerations
Advantages
- able to be performed with cataract surgery or separately
- may induce less postoperative healing time, glare, and discomfort than corneal relaxing incisions (CRIs) because the incision is placed at the limbus instead of inside the cornea
- a practical, relatively simple, and forgiving way to correct astigmatism (axis placement and the length of the incisions not critically precise regarding refractive effect)
- rare overcorrections

Indications
- visually significant cataracts and 0.50 to 3.00 D of astigmatism
- strong patient desire for diminished or eliminated dependency on spectacles or contact lenses following cataract surgery
- candidates for clear lens extraction who have up to 3.00 D of astigmatism

Surgical Considerations
Equipment
- corneal topographer and keratometer (determines the amount, axis, and symmetry of corneal cylinder)
- a marking device (mark the steep axis determined by topography)
- a surgical keratometer (confirms axis results before placing incisions)
- an RK/AK surgical diamond knife (e.g., the Lab Instruments L320 micrometer knife)

Methods
- For phakic patients more than 73 years old
  - Customize LRI placement according to topography. (Do not consider refractive cylinder.)
  - For asymmetric astigmatism, elongate the LRI slightly in the steepest of the two steep axes and shorten it (by the same slight amount) in the flatter of the two steep axes.
  - For nonorthogonal astigmatism, place each of the paired LRIs at the steepest portion of the topography "bow tie" that was indicated by topography (i.e., you do not need to create paired LRIs in the same meridian).
  - Mark the steep meridian of astigmatism with cautery based on the topography results that were confirmed with surgical keratometry.
  - Using the diamond knife (set at 600 μm for most cases), place a 6-mm incision on the steep axis at the limbus barely anterior to the palisades of Vogt (for 1.00 D, use one 6-mm incision; for 1.00–2.00 D, use two 6-mm incisions; for 2.00–3.00 D, use two 8-mm incisions).
- Make shorter incisions for phakic patients less than 73 years old to achieve the same refractive effect as for older patients.
- For patients older than 80 years or those who have corneoscleral thinning, use a diamond blade set at 500 μm.
- For pseudophakic patients
  - Use the same nomogram as for phakic patients.
  - Base axis and amount of astigmatism on refraction *only*.
  - Base the steep meridian on *only* the axis of refractive cylinder.
  - Determine the symmetry of astigmatism using topography only.

Postoperative Considerations
Complications
- limbal bleeding from limbal vessels
- undercorrection
- perforation (rare)

Enhancements

- If a single 6-mm LRI results in undercorrection, extend the incisions to 8 mm, or make a second 6-mm incision.
- If you have made two 8-mm incisions but undercorrection still exists, then perform CRIs to treat the residual astigmatism (also for initial astigmatism >3.00 D with LRI).
- For corneal relaxing incisions (more likely to produce glare and discomfort than are LRIs because they are placed inside the corneal limbus)
  - First, place two 8-mm LRIs on the steep axis at the limbus.
  - Set the diamond blade at 99% of corneal depth (as determined by pachymetry).
  - Create one 2-mm incision for every diopter of astigmatism over 3 D and allow an 8-mm OZ. (Exact axial placement of CRIs along the steep axis is critical because CRIs produce significantly more refractive effect than do LRIs.)

Suggested Readings

Assil KK, Schanzlin DJ. *Radial and Astigmatic Keratotomy: A Complete Handbook.* St. Louis, MO: Poole Press; 1994.

Gills JP. *Nomogram for Limbal Relaxing Incisions with Cataract Surgery.* Tarpon Springs, FL: St Luke's Cataract and Laser Institute; 1999.

Sanders DR, Hofmann RF. *Refractive Surgery: A Text of Radial Keratotomy.* Thorofare, NJ: Slack Inc.; 1980.

CHAPTER 9

Photorefractive Keratectomy

Mihai Pop

CHAPTER CONTENTS

PREOPERATIVE CONSIDERATIONS

Indications
• recurrent corneal erosion
• Reis-Bücklers dystrophy
• map-dot fingerprint or stromal corneal dystrophies (e.g., granular, macular, or lattice dystrophies)
• keratoconus (specific cases with stable refraction, limited astigmatism, and normal pachymetry)
• laser adjustment after keratoplasty, clear lens extraction, or cataract extraction

Inclusion Criteria
• realistic patient expectations
• clinically normal eyes
• patient age greater than 18 years (required for refractive stability)
• postoperative pachymetry not less than 300 μm (ablation depths calculated preoperatively)
• postoperative keratometry not less than 36 D (ablation depths calculated preoperatively)
• scotopic pupil size less than 8 mm for an excimer laser [provides an optical zone

(OZ) <6 mm with no transition zone capability]
• good general health (patients with diabetes or HIV treatable if health permits but do not perform simultaneous bilateral surgery; see Contraindications)

Patient Evaluation
• manifest refraction
• measurement of best-corrected visual acuity (BCVA) using Snellen's charts
• evaluation of pupil size in scotopic conditions using a Colvard pupillometer (model no. 0401; Oasis Medical)
• corneal topography
• slit-lamp examination of anterior segment
• fundus eye examination (for myopia >5 D)
• assessment of contrast sensitivity visual acuity under controlled luminance
• evaluation of halos or glare
  ○ Hold an Amsler grid 6 ft from the patient.
  ○ Project a single, light dot at the center of the grid.
  ○ Ask the patient to indicate with a laser pointer the regions where halos or glare occur.
  ○ Draw halos and glare on the grid.

Patient Preparation

- Instruct patient to remove soft contact lenses 2 to 3 days before the preoperative examination.
- For rigid gas-permeable contact lens wearers, verify the stability of topography before surgery (stability may take 4–6 weeks to occur).

SURGICAL CONSIDERATIONS

Contraindications

- relative contraindications
  - scotopic pupil size greater than 8 mm (greater risk of having postoperative glare and halos)
  - human immunodeficiency virus (HIV) (depends on general health status)
  - diabetes (depends on general health status)
  - infections that call for surgery to be delayed (e.g., a common cold, sinusitis, and other infectious illnesses)
  - ocular pathology (especially autoimmune disease)
  - dry-eye syndrome [often associated with systemic diseases such as sarcoidosis, mucin deficiency (e.g., Stevens-Johnson syndrome), avitaminose A, lipid deficiency (blepharitis), and decreased blinking (from contact lens use and post–herpes simplex keratitis)]
- absolute contraindications
  - unrealistic patient expectations about surgical "guarantees" (e.g., that surgery will not harm vision, the outcome will be plano, or spectacles or contacts will no longer be necessary)
  - unstable or progressive myopia or hyperopia
  - amblyopia or strabismus (inform patients with very low fusional amplitudes that the procedure will not improve their BCVA)

General Methods

- Calibrate the laser for the exact ablation rate according to the excimer laser manufacturer's directions.
- Give an oral analgesic to the patient 15 to 30 min before surgery.
- Instill 1 or 2 drops of ofloxacin 0.3% drops (Floxin or Ocuflox) 5 min before and 1 to 2 drops seconds before insertion of lid speculum.
- Instill 1 or 2 drops of 0.5% proparacaine hydrochloride (Alcaine or Ophthaine) 15 min before and a few more drops seconds before lid speculum insertion.
- Anesthetize the cornea and surrounding tissues, including the palpebral conjunctiva and edge of the eyelid, with a soaked cotton swab of 0.5% proparacaine hydrochloride.
- Place the head of the patient in the supine position with the chin higher than the forehead as you look into the microscope (rotate the patient's head with your hands if needed).
- Insert lid speculum.
- Because the upper eyelid may push debris into the ablation zone, you should be able to see the upper part of the limbus under the speculum (debris and tear stream are evacuated toward the upper limbus by microblinking the eye).
- Prevent eyelashes from entering the path of the laser beam with tape, if necessary.
- Carefully dry the conjunctival sac (cul-de-sac) (a potential hazard for infection).
- Perform epithelial debridement with an Amoils epithelial scrubber or laser transepithelial removal.
- Gently wipe away any remaining epithelial debris with an eye spear.
- Absorb all excess fluid with a sponge.
- Determine the total amount of myopia and astigmatism to correct using a laser-specific nomogram and your own experience.

- Perform multipasses to divide the total treatment by specific nomograms (see Nomograms).
- Do not exceed 20 sec per division for laser treatment.
- Cool the cornea by adding chilled balanced saline solution (BSS).
- Administer medications immediately after the procedure.
  ○ 2 drops of 0.5% ketorolac tromethamine (Acular)
  ○ 2 drops of 0.3% ofloxacin
- Place a soft disposable contact lens on the eye (Fig. 9–1).
- Instruct the patient to wear sunglasses as protection from ultraviolet (UV) light.
- Ensure the quality of the sunglasses for blocking UV light.

Nomograms

THE MULTIZONE AND MULTIPASS TECHNIQUE The first multizone technique for PRK was developed to decrease the ablation depth for broad-beam excimer lasers. Later, the multizone/multipass

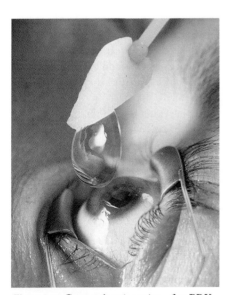

Figure 9–1 Contact lens insertion after PRK.

technique was designed for use with these lasers to improve refractive results.

Methods
- initial pretreatment at a 2.5-mm diameter of 1.0 or 1.5 D (depending on the degree of myopia)
- division of remainder of treatment into several small corrections or passes between 3.5 and 6.0 mm in diameter
- correction of an equal amount of sphere at the same laser pass
- performance of cylinder correction at a diameter of 5.0 mm*
- stoppage of broad-beam laser and resetting of diaphragm to zero between subtreatments
- performance of multiple passes over the same OZ
- a slight shifting of zones
  ○ a smoother ablated surface with fewer ridges on the ablated surface
  ○ smoother concentric steps
  ○ less potential for tissue deposits
- laser diaphragm (increases in size during the treatment and delimits zones)
- smaller treatments
  ○ use of a specific algorithm titrated to the level of myopia (low to moderate)
  ○ each ablative pass (≤ 7 total) lasts 10 to 30 sec
- treatment of astigmatism with an elliptical ablation combined with multizone/multipass ablations

THE SCANNING MULTIPASS TECHNIQUE This technique is derived from the initial multizone/multipass technique and may be used with a scanning laser [e.g., Bausch and Lomb (Rochester, NY) 217 laser or Laser-Sight LSX].

*See Pop and Aras (1995) for a description of multizone/multipass algorithms.

Advantages

- use for low to high myopia or hyperopia (use laser- and surgeon-specific nomograms to adjust the total amount of myopia and astigmatism to correct by determining the fixed ratio that indicates the coefficient to apply to actual sphere and cylinder to obtain the desired sphere and cylinder corrections)
- no need for pretreatment for central island
- use of 6-mm OZ with a transition zone of 9 mm (large transitional zones are used to smooth the curve between the actual treatment zone and the remaining untouched corneal stroma)
- elimination of the need to perform multizones
  ○ generation of multiple scanning of the corneal surface while removing stroma
  ○ performance of equal passes so that the initial sphere is divided by equal but smaller treatments (sum of small treatments equals target correction)
  ○ introduction of very small rest periods between subtreatments
  ○ decreased haze for high myopes
- passes (≤ 6 total) should each last 20 to 30 sec (do not exceed 30 sec per pass)
- no need to wet the surface between passes

Disadvantages

- potential for calculation errors (if not automated)
- dehydration of corneal stromal (if excessive time between passes causing overcorrection)

Myopia

Equipment Preparation

- Configure the laser to treat all astigmatism (generally, 10–30% is removed from the computed sphere; may vary with different types and brands of lasers).

Nomogram

- patients less than 40 years old
  ○ removal of 0.25 D of astigmatism to the computed sphere per diopter of cylinder

[e.g., $-6.00 - 1.00 \times 45$ degrees $= 30\%$ (2 D) and $+0.25$ D removed to the sphere; because of 1 D of cylinder; the computed ablation $= -3.75 - 1.00 \times 45$ degrees)

- patients greater than 40 years old
  ○ removal of an additional 0.25 D to the computed sphere

Results

- myopia less than 4 D
  ○ 97% of eyes within ± 1 D of emmetropia
  ○ 4% needing retreatment
  ○ no eyes with clinically significant haze
  ○ no eyes with loss of more than 1 line of BCVA
- myopia from 4 to 8 D
  ○ 95% of eyes within ± 1 D of emmetropia
  ○ 9% needing retreatment
  ○ 0.2% of eyes with mild to moderate haze
  ○ no eyes with loss of more than 1 line of BCVA
- myopia from 8 to 10 D
  ○ 83% of eyes within ± 1 D of emmetropia
  ○ 12% needing retreatment
  ○ 2% of eyes with mild to moderate haze
  ○ 0.6% of eyes with loss of more than 1 line of BCVA
- myopia greater than 10 D
  ○ 80% of eyes within ± 1D of emmetropia
  ○ 14% needing retreatment
  ○ 2% of eyes with mild to moderate haze
  ○ 1.4% of eyes with loss of more than 1 line of BCVA
- equal results 1 month after surgery with photorefractive keratectomy (PRK) or laser in situ keratomileusis (LASIK) for myopia less than 10 D (Fig. 9–2)

Hyperopia

Equipment Preparation

- Set the slit-scanning laser to a repetition rate of 41 Hz with a polymethylmetha-

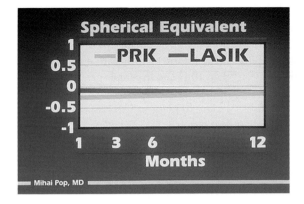

Figure 9–2 Postoperative comparison of PRK and LASIK spherical equivalents for myopia <10 D. No significant refractive outcome differences are found 1 month after surgery.

crylate/cornea ratio of 1.0 and a cylinder/sphere time rate of 0.45 (observe ~12 sec/D of correction).

Results
- hyperopia less than +3 D
  - 92% of eyes within ±1 D of emmetropia
  - 8% needing retreatment
  - 3% of eyes with mild to moderate haze
  - regression of +0.75 to +1 D
  - 2% of eyes with loss of more than 1 line of BCVA

Compound Astigmatism
Methods
- Perform a cross-cylinder technique using Vinciguerra's nomogram for astigmatism greater than 3 D (see Vinciguerra et al., 1999).

- Dividing the astigmatism in two treatments.
- Perform half of the cylinder in minus cylinder and the other half in plus cylinder (e.g., the treatment of −4.00 − 6.00 × 180 degrees would be plano +3.00 × 90 degrees, plano −3.00 × 180 degrees, and −7.00 D total spherical ablation).
- removal of 0.25 D of astigmatism to the sphere per diopter of cylinder (see Myopia)

Mixed Astigmatism
Methods
- Use Chayet's nomogram (Table 9–1).
- Use cylindrical correction with both myopic and hyperopic cylinder modes of the laser to split the amount of ablation made to the steep and flat meridians of an astigmatic cornea.

TABLE 9–1

Chayet's Astigmatism Nomogram

	Meridians	
	Flat	Steep
Simple myopic astigmatism		
−1.0 D spherical component	7%–16%	84%–93%
0.0 D spherical component	25%	75%
Mixed astigmatism		
0.0 D spherical equivalent	63%	37%
+1.0 D spherical equivalent	80%	20%
Simple hyperopic astigmatism	100%	0%

- Perform only a portion of the steep meridian correction and a portion of the flat meridian correction [elliptical ablation in the steep meridian (myopic astigmatism) results in a hyperopic shift].
- Assume that ablation in the steep meridian always induces a 33% hyperopic shift, never to exceed 30% of the cylindrical component.
  - For example, $+2.00 - 4.00 \times 0$ degrees $= 0.37\%$ of -4 D is plano -1.5×0 degrees, which is corrected on the steep meridian ablation.
  - After inducing 33% of hyperopic shift, the refraction is $+2.50 - 2.50 \times 0$ degrees, which can be translated to plano $+2.50 \times 90$ degrees that can be corrected on the flat meridian ablation.
- Do not confuse which axis is to be targeted for which ablation.
- Begin with the minus cylinder.

Presbyopia
Patient Preparation
- Try monovision with contact lenses before proceeding with surgery (if the patient feels comfortable with this vision, proceed with the procedure).

Methods
- Although monovision is the only alternative to PRK for improvement of near vision, it is not considered real correction of accommodation.
  - Correct one eye, usually the dominant one, toward emmetropia.
  - Undercorrect the other eye with a slight level of myopia (-0.50 to -1.50 D).

Alternative Treatments
LASER IN SITU KERATOMILEUSIS The upper limit for PRK may be between -7 and -12 D. For severe myopia (> -12 D), predictability decreases but the incidence of certain adverse effects (e.g., corneal haze) significantly increases to greater than 10% from less than 1% for low myopia corrections. Inform patients with myopia greater than 10 D and hyperopia greater than 3 D of the greater risks associated with the procedure (60% of patients experience excellent results).

- retreatments
- halos
- haze
- loss of BCVA

PHAKIC INTRAOCULAR LENS INSERTION Implant a phakic anterior chamber intraocular lens (IOL) in patients with myopia greater than 10 D or hyperopia greater than 3 D if the anterior chamber depth and axial length allow such an invasive procedure (see Chapters 14 and 16).

CLEAR LENSECTOMY Perform clear lensectomy with a posterior chamber IOL for patients with presbyopia. If the exact intended correction is not achieved after insertion of an IOL or a phakic IOL, retreatment can be performed with PRK or LASIK (see Retreatment).

HOLIUM LASER KERATOPLASTY This can be used to treat low hyperopia (<2.5 D).

POSTOPERATIVE CONSIDERATIONS

Medications
- corticosteroids [reverse inflammatory reaction but the mechanism of corticosteroids on keratocytes is still unclear and may cause increased intraocular pressure (IOP) or cataracts]
  - Administer 0.1% fluorometholone (Eflone, Flarex, Fluor-Op) 1 to 2 drops

every 4 hr for the first day and then 3 times a day for the next 48 hr.

○ Use topical corticosteroids (see above) for the first 4 to 5 months (depends on the healing of the cornea for patients with myopia >5 D or hyperopia)

○ Increase the dosage of topical corticosteroids at the second month and then taper by 1 drop per day per month (most of the inflammatory reaction peaks near the second month after surgery).

○ Prescribe topical 0.1% fluorometholone to patients with myopia greater than 5 D (2 times a day for the first postoperative month, 4 times a day for the second month, 3 times a day for the third month, 2 times a day for the fourth month, and 1 time a day for the fifth month).

○ Prescribe 0.1% fluorometholone for patients with myopia less than 5 D (3 times a day only during the first week after surgery).

○ Consider prompt retreatment before increasing the corticosteroid regimen for patients with increasing haze (advanced haze formation can activate mechanisms that can create further haze even after retreatment; see Retreatment).

• antibiotics
○ Prescribe a consistent regimen to reduce the risk of infection (start medication a few hours after surgery).

○ Instill 0.3% ofloxacin every 4 hr for the first 72 hr and 3 times a day for the following week (the kill curve is ~3 hr, at which time 99.9% of bactericidal concentration is attained for Gram-positive bacteria, including *Staphylococcus aureus, S. epidermidis,* and *S. pneumoniae* and Gram-negative bacteria such as *Haemophilus influenzae*).

• artificial tears
○ Prescribe 4 times a day for 1 to 3 months after surgery (mandatory and greatly helps the healing process and patient comfort)

• oral analgesics (for pain management during the first 72 hr of re-epithelialization)

• Give nonsteroidal anti-inflammatory drugs (NSAIDs; 0.5% ketorolac tromethamine) every 4 hr for the first day and 3 times a day for the next 48 hr.

Complications

• loss of BCVA
○ often the result of haze
○ after prompt retreatment, lines of visual acuity regained

• undercorrection or overcorrection without haze
○ Plan prompt retreatment as early as 1 month after surgery.
○ Stop corticosteroids 2 to 3 days before retreatment.

• epithelial or stromal haze
○ graded on a scale of 0 to 5 (Table 9–2)
○ avoid by using an epithelial brush, chilled BSS after surgery, planned corticotherapy, and sunglasses to protect the eyes from UV light
○ risk decreased by using the multizone/multipass technique (Fig. 9–3)
○ generally increases near the second month after surgery and then decreases
○ decreases with use of scanning excimer lasers

• halos, glare, and starburst (Fig. 9–4)
○ caused by the pupil dilating to a greater diameter than the treatment optical zone (OZ)
○ incidence greatly decreased by OZs greater than 4 mm and transition zones
○ Stiles-Crawford effect (a spherical aberration of retinal directional sensitivity caused by the effect of light passing through the center of the pupil; insignificant for pupil size >4 mm and peaks for 8-mm pupil size)

TABLE 9–2

Grades of Haze

Grade	Description
0	Clear cornea, with a possibility of a very light haze. There is no difference in texture between the central treated zone and the peripheral nontreated zone. The normal corneal stroma has a ground glass appearance.
0.25	Trace haze is defined as faint corneal haze just perceptible by broad oblique illumination. It is the minimal amount of corneal haze present in the grading scale and is characterized by a diffuse "cotton floss" appearance of the corneal stroma.
0.5	The haze is faint when seen by broad oblique illumination and is comparable to a light cottony cloud in the stroma. Although more perceptible than 0.25 trace haze, neither 0.25 nor 0.5 haze can be identified with broad direct illumination.
1.0	The haze is difficult to see by direct focal slit illumination. It is easier to see than the 0.5 faint haze by broad oblique illumination. The cottony cloud is more intense.
2.0	Haze affecting lightly the refraction: it is hardly seen by direct focal slit illumination. By broad oblique illumination, it has a more granular aspect than 1.0 haze.
3.0	Moderate haze: refraction is possible but with difficulty. It is considered as a moderately dense opacity that partially obscures the iris in direct illumination. Frequently, the haze is scattered in a series of small dots.
4.0	The opacity affects completely the refraction: the anterior chamber can be seen. The haze obscures any details of the iris. It is the first grade able to be seen without using any instrument. In direct slit illumination, it is a white-gray corneal opacity that may display thickness and elevation. Extremely rare.
5.0	The opacity makes the examination of the anterior chamber difficult or impossible. Almost never seen.

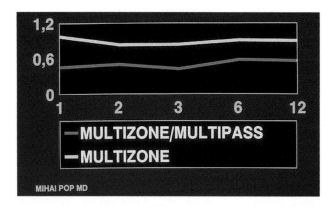

Figure 9–3 Comparison of mean haze for multizone and multizone/multipass PRK for myopia (1–20 D) using a broad-beam laser. Multizone/multipass PRK significantly decreases the amount of postoperative haze.

- ○ may be decreased someday by wavefront technology (accounts for the optical dry eye; see Chapter 12)
- ○ usually resolves within 6 to 12 months of surgery

- • dry eye
  - ○ Perform a Schirmer's test and verify tear break-up time or ocular surface with dye staining pattern.
  - ○ Prescribe artificial tears without preser-

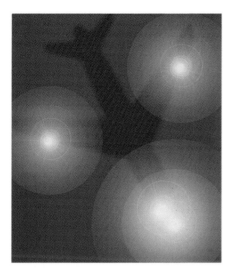

Figure 9–4 An artist's depiction of halos.

vatives [newly developed artificial tears, such as TheraTears (Advanced Vision Research Inc., Woburn, MA) have balanced electrolytes that are more suitable for the eye].

◦ Use punctum plugs for extreme cases.
• severe bilateral complication (incidence theoretically estimated at 0.01%)
• secondary effects from medications (check for increased IOP with corticosteroid use)
• sterile infiltrates (if present within the first few postoperative days, discontinue NSAIDs, remove the contact lens immediately, and patch the eye if re-epithelialization is not complete)

RETREATMENT

Identification and classification of patients who require retreatment are subtle because some patients with mild corrections or haze are symptomatic whereas others are completely satisfied with their outcome.

Indications
• corneal haze
  ◦ Early diagnosis is mandatory.

◦ Retreatments are possible as early as 1 month after surgery before haze formation increases.
◦ Avoid severe haze by retreating promptly (advanced haze formation can activate mechanisms that create further haze even after retreatment).
◦ Retreatment of eyes with an aggressive healing pattern that is accompanied by a progressive myopic shift may create the same amount of haze when performed 6 to 12 months after the original treatment.
• undercorrections, overcorrections, and regression
  ◦ These are correctable within 1 to 4 months after surgery.
  ◦ Stable refractive outcomes may result from prompt retreatment.
  ◦ Use holmium laser keratoplasty for overcorrections less than +1.50 D.

Results
• up to 95% of eyes within ±1 D
• possibility of lost lines of BCVA after retreatment

Phototherapeuthic Keratectomy
Methods
• Perform phototherapeutic keratectomy (PTK) under low light intensity of the laser microscope to see the epithelial pseudofluorescence.
• Remove the epithelium by setting the laser to a depth of 55 μm for the optical and transition zone diameters.
• Stop the laser as soon as you see a black ring disturbing the pseudofluorescence of the epithelium.
• Remove any residual epithelial cell layer manually.
  ◦ very easy for minimal or no haze
  ◦ not recommended for moderate to severe haze (epithelial debris and cells remain between the island of scarred tissue that

makes an irregular surface before retreatment; may result in unpredictable outcomes and increased chances of secondary scarring; use transepithelial PTK)

- Proceed with usual algorithms for treatment of the refractive error as previously described.
- Retreat refraction of patients with haze (very rare in patients with <6 D of myopia).
- For advanced haze, treat only half the refraction because overcorrection may occur (initial manifest refraction may be imprecise; Fig. 9–5).

PHOTOTHERAPEUTIC KERATECTOMY AFTER RADIAL KERATECTOMY

Indications

- management of the small ridges usually found over the radial keratectomy (RK) incisions (found under the epithelium as the result of the stroma reaction following RK; retreatment is vital)

Methods

- Perform PTK at 6.0 mm diameter with a stromal depth of 70 μm to eliminate the small RK ridges.
- Stop PTK before reaching 70 μm (PTK may provide uniformity and homogeneity on the stromal surface).

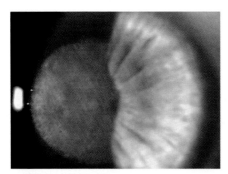

Figure 9–5 Advanced (grade 3) haze following PRK. BCVA decreased to 20/200.

- Maintain PTK until the loss of pseudofluorescence over the ridges is about 1.5 to 2.0 mm wide.
- When the nonfluorescent area on the incisions appears and is ±1 mm wide, stop and treat the residual myopia (proceeding creates depressions along the RK incisions).
- After removing RK incision ridges, manually clean the remaining epithelium and perform PRK treatment as usual using the manifest refraction evaluated before surgery.
- Keep OZ at 5.0 to 5.5 mm (an OZ of 6.0 mm is not necessary because RK has already provided a relative transition zone for PRK).
- If inexperienced, stop the treatment every 10 sec and ask the patient to fixate on the aiming diode, recenter the pupil, and resume the procedure.
- Control patient eye movement by positioning your hands to recenter the treatment (one hand on the patient's forehead and the other hand on the focusing mechanism of the laser or use an eyetracker device to aim the laser).
- Indicate to the patient how many seconds of the treatment remain every 5 to 10 sec.
- Reassure the patient that everything is going well to ensure patient cooperation.
- Cool the cornea with chilled (4°C) BSS.
- After treatment, instill antibiotic drops to prevent infection and wash out debris.
- Do *not* wipe the cornea with a microsurgical sponge (small particles may catch under the contact lens and cause patient discomfort).
- Manipulate the outer surface of the contact lens carefully with a soaked microsurgical sponge to avoid contact with the inner surface and the introduction of foreign body material or debris.
- Do not use forceps because they may damage the surface of the contact lens.

Postoperative Care

- Examine the patient's eyes 72 hr after surgery or daily until reepithelialization and at 1, 2, 3, 6, 12, and 24 months (for lower myopes, omit 2- and 6-month follow-ups if the patient's condition does not change).
  - Perform manifest refraction.
- Evaluate patient's BCVA and uncorrected visual acuity using a Snellen's chart.
  - Use corneal topography to check for increased astigmatism or irregular astigmatism.
  - Grade haze on a scale of 0 to 3 (clear to completely obscured), as proposed by some authors.
- After correcting for astigmatism with PRK, perform a vector analysis on preoperative refraction rather than postoperative refraction.
- To estimate the quality of astigmatic correction, calculate Alpin's index of success (defined as the proportion of the remaining astigmatism to treat on the corneal plane divided by the intended correction) using medical computer software.
- Analyze refractive outcomes and, if needed, adjust excimer laser nomograms (computer software packages, such as the ASSORT Eye Surgery Analysis Program from the Melbourne Excimer Group in Melbourne, Australia, may help in this task).

Suggested Readings

Griffith M, Jackson BW, Lafontaine MD, Mintsioulis G, Agapitos P, Hodge W. Evaluation of current techniques of corneal epithelial removal in hyperopic photorefractive keratectomy. *J Cataract Refract Surg.* 1998;24:1070–1078.

Jackson BW, Casson E, Hodge W, Mintsioulis G, Agapitos PJ. Laser vision correction for low hyperopia. *Ophthalmology.* 1998;105:1727–1738.

Kim JH, Hahn TW, Young CL. Photorefractive keratectomy in 202 myopic eyes: one year results. *Refract Corneal Surg.* 1993;9(suppl): S11–S16.

Kitazawa Y, Tokoro T, Ito S, Ishii Y. The efficacy of cooling on excimer laser photorefractive keratectomy in the rabbit eye. *Survey Ophthalmol.* 1997;42(Suppl 1):S82–S88.

O'Brart DP, Lohmann CP, Fitze FW, Smith SE, Kerr-Muir MG, Marshall J. Night vision after excimer laser photorefractive keratectomy: haze and halos. *Eur J Ophthalmol.* 1994;4:43–51.

Pop M. Prompt retreatment after photorefractive keratectomy. *J Cataract Refract Surg.* 1998; 24:320–326.

Pop M, Aras M. Multizone/multipass photorefractive keratectomy: six months results. *J Cataract Refract Surg.* 1995;21:633–643.

Pop M, Payette Y. Multipass versus single pass photorefractive keratectomy for high myopia using a scanning laser. *J Refract Surg.* 1999;15: 444–450.

Pop M, Payette Y. Results of bilateral photorefractive keratectomy. *Ophthalmology.* 2000;107: 472–479.

Vinciguerra P, Epstein D, Azzolini M, Radice P, Sborgia M. Algorithm to correct hyperopic astigmatism with the Nidek EC-5000 excimer laser. *J Refract Surg.* 1999;15(suppl):S186–S187.

CHAPTER 10

Laser Thermal Keratoplasty

Abdelmonem M. Hamed and Douglas D. Koch

CHAPTER CONTENTS

The Holmium:Yttrium-Aluminum-Garnet
Laser

Future Directions

Suggested Readings

In 1898, the Dutch medical student Leendert Lans demonstrated that localized heating with electrocautery can change the curvature of a rabbit cornea by inducing thermal shrinkage of collagen fibers. In 1964, Stringer and Parr reported that the shrinkage temperature of corneal collagen was 55 to 58°C. Gasset and Kaufman clinically applied thermal keratoplasty with a heated metal probe in 1975. Neumann et al described radial thermal keratoplasty in 1990, which proved to be of little value because of the high incidence of regression and poor predictability of results. Despite extensive study using several devices and technologies, investigators have abandoned most nonlaser modalities because of many problems:
• poor refractive predictability
• delayed epithelial healing
• recurrent corneal erosions (RCEs)
• corneal neovascularization and scarring
• regression
• stromal necrosis
• iritis
• corneal endothelial decompensation

Fortunately, computer-controlled laser technology for thermal keratoplasty enables surgeons to deliver controlled quantities of light energy to heat the cornea with exquisite precision but minimal damage to surrounding tissue. Several laser modalities are potential choices for performing laser thermal keratoplasty (LTK), of which holmium:yttrium-aluminum-garnet (Ho:YAG) is the most popular:
• Ho:YAG lasers
• diode lasers
• erbium lasers
• carbon-dioxide lasers

In this chapter, we review the advances, clinical applications, limitations, and future directions of Ho:YAG LTK.

THE HOLMIUM:YTTRIUM-ALUMINUM-GARNET LASER

The Ho:YAG laser is a solid-state laser that emits radiation in the infrared region of the electromagnetic spectrum. The anterior corneal stroma primarily absorbs the laser beam, which creates a cone-shaped temperature profile.

Advantages
- adjustability of pulse duration, repetition rate, energy per pulse, and number of pulses (achieves the ideal temperature elevation to optimize collagen shrinkage without overheating the cornea)
- ideal penetration depth (480–530 μm) for achieving stromal heating with minimal damage to adjacent tissue (no clinical data demonstrate superior long-term stability with deeper penetration)
- better refractive corrections and better long-term stability (because of more pronounced shrinkage of collagen fibrils in the anterior stroma than in the posterior stroma created by the cone-shaped stromal temperature profile vs. the cylinder-like profile produced by the hot needle used for radial thermal keratoplasty)
- ability to perform additional treatments or enhancements on patients with residual hyperopia after initial Ho:YAG LTK treatments
- usefulness for treating myopes who have been overcorrected by PRK or LASIK

Indications
- low to moderate hyperopia (+0.75–+3.0 D)
- refractive and keratometric astigmatism less than 1.0 D

Inclusion Criteria
- patient age more than 40 years
- best corrected visual acuity (BCVA) of 20/40 or better in both eyes
- normal intraocular pressure (10–20 mmHg)
- normal corneal thickness (490–590 μm)
- stable refraction for 12 months before surgery

- no history of corneal surgery or trauma (except for previous excimer laser corneal surgery)
- no ocular pathology (e.g., corneal diseases, glaucoma, or cataracts)
- no history of systemic steroid, antimetabolite, or immunosuppressant use

Two main Ho:YAG laser delivery systems have been investigated: a contact device and a noncontact device, each of which produces a different corneal temperature-time-space distribution. Generalize carefully about results obtained with various devices because differences in any of the many treatment parameters may dramatically affect the device's thermal effects on the cornea.

Contact Laser Thermal Keratoplasty
Summit Technology Inc. (Waltham, MA) developed the first contact-probe Ho:YAG laser, which emits electromagnetic radiation and has the following specifications.

Laser Specifications
- 2.06-μm wavelength
- 300-msec pulses
- frequency of 15 Hz
- a quartz fiberoptic handpiece (delivers energy to the corneal stroma)
- a sapphire tip that has a cone angle of 120 degrees (focuses the laser energy to form a wedge-shaped collagen shrinkage zone that measures 700 μm in diameter at the corneal surface and a depth of approximately 450 μm) (Fig. 10–1)

Advantages
- ability to heat stromal collagen to a higher average temperature compared with a noncontact device
  - delivers approximately twice as much energy per spot (19 mJ × 25 pulses vs. 24–30 mJ × 10 pulses)

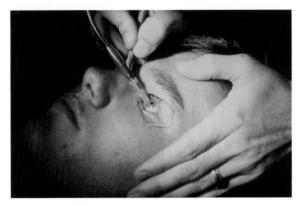

Figure 10–1 The contact holmium energy is focused with a sapphire tip that has a cone angle of 120 degrees.

◦ has three times the pulse repetition frequency (15 vs. 5 Hz)

◦ delivers a higher irradiance (strongly vs. weakly focused) geometry

Methods*

• Administer topical anesthesia and 1% pilocarpine preoperatively.

• Mark the cornea with a marking instrument to define probe placements.

• Apply the contact focusing tip to the corneal surface in a consistent manner to minimize induction of irregular astigmatism.

Results†

• successful reduction of hyperopia (mean correction of 1.13 D in four patients at 1 year and 1.63 D in two patients at 2 years)

• stabilization of most regression by 6 months (continuation of regression documented in patients followed for 3 years)

*These methods are for the Summit device; presumably, the Technomed unit (Baesweiler, Germany), which is being investigated in Europe uses analogous procedures.

†These are results of the Summit laser phase II trial (see Yanoff, 1995, and Thompson, 1994 in Suggested Readings).

• negligible incidence of induced astigmatism at 1 year

• identification of need for further refinement of predictability of the achieved correction

• abandonment of study because of 3-year regression findings

Noncontact Laser Thermal Keratoplasty

Noncontact Ho:YAG LTK uses a slit-lamp delivery system (the Corneal Shaping System) from Sunrise Technologies (Fremont, CA) that does not touch the corneal surface.

Laser Specifications

• laser wavelength of 2.13 μm

• a pulse duration of 250 μs (full width at half of maximum intensity)

• a pulse repetition frequency of 5 Hz

• an adjustable pulse energy up to 300 mJ (24–30 mJ × 10 pulses)

• projection of a ring pattern (3–8 mm wide) of up to eight spots on the cornea (some studies have used one to three rings with inner-ring diameters as small as 5 mm)

• nominal spot diameter of 600 μm (containing 90% of the energy per spot)

• a nonuniform energy density distribution within the spot

REFRACTIVE SURGERY: A COLOR SYNOPSIS

Advantages
• well-tolerated by patients
• little maintenance
• safety
• ease of use

Indications
• hyperopia to 2.5 D

Methods
• Center treatments along the line of sight by centering the red helium neon (HeNe) laser tracer beams (wavelength = 633 nm) around the entrance pupil while the patient views a red light-emitting diode fixation source.
• Focus the laser on the surface of the cornea using calibrated green HeNe laser-focusing beams (wavelength = 543 nm).
• Begin administering topical anesthesia at least 10 min prior to treatment (1 drop at 5-min intervals up to a total of 4 drops).
• Introduce a lid speculum to open the eyelids 5 min after administering the last anesthetic drop.
• Hold the eyelids open for 3 min to allow the tear film to dry before beginning treatment.
  ○ Because water absorbs the laser light, the timing of drops and tear-film drying is designed to standardize epithelial swelling and corneal hydration and to maximize evaporation of the tear film.
• Deliver 5 to 10 laser pulses to each treatment ring sequentially over 1 to 2 sec with total treatment energy of 2.1 to 2.4 J per ring.
• Administer antibiotic and nonsteroidal anti-inflammatory drops four times a day until the epithelium heals (usually 1–2 days).

CLINICAL STUDIES Safety and efficacy trials with the Sunrise device began outside the United States in 1993. Results from four clinical studies have been reported. In each of these trials, none of the treated eyes lost two or more lines of BCVA, and there were no clinically significant complications.

Study Parameters and Results
• Koch et al (the first sighted-eye study to correct low hyperopia ≤ 3 D)
  ○ 15 patients (1 eye each)
  ○ one ring of eight spots
  ○ centerline diameter of 6 mm
  ○ 10 pulses of 159 to 199 mJ
  ○ follow-up at 2 years
  ○ improved mean uncorrected visual acuity (UCVA) (from 20/125-1 to 20/50-2)
  ○ mean refractive correction of −1.1 D (−0.38 to −2.63 D) for 11 eyes (73%)
  ○ no persistent refractive correction (±0.25D) for four eyes (27%)
  ○ mean induced refractive astigmatism of 0.18 D
  ○ 2.0 D of regression between 6 months and 2 years on average
• Kohnen et al
  ○ 39 eyes with up to +4.75 D of hyperopia
  ○ treated with two rings of eight spots each
  ○ radial spot patterns of 5 and 6 mm, 6 and 7 mm, or 6.5 and 7.5 mm (groups A, B, and C)
  ○ fixed pulse energy of 240 mJ
  ○ 5 pulses of laser light administered per ring
  ○ mean increases in lines of UCVA at 1 year for groups A, B, and C (3.7 ± 0.5, 6.8 ± 2.7, and 5.3 ± 3.3, respectively)
  ○ mean change in the spherical equivalent of the manifest refraction (−2.08 ± 1.13 D, −1.83 ± 0.88 D, −1.22 ± 0.88 D, respectively)
  ○ good refractive stability after 6 months
• Koch et al, 1997 [phase IIa U.S. Food and Drug Administration (FDA) trials of noncontact Ho:YAG LTK]
  ○ 28 eyes with up to +3.88 D of hyperopia

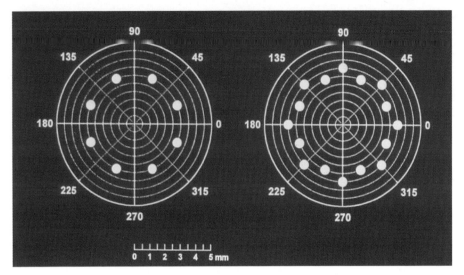

Figure 10–2 One- and two-ring patterns used in early noncontact Ho:YAG LTK studies.

- ○ one or two rings each containing eight spots
- ○ centerline diameters of 6 mm (one ring) or 6 to 7 mm (two rings) (Fig. 10–2)
- ○ 10 pulses of 208 to 242 mJ
- ○ improved UCVA by one or more lines in 19 of 26 (73%) of the treated eyes at 2 years
- ○ mean change in spherical equivalent of the subjective manifest refraction (−0.53 ± 0.33 D and −1.48 ± 0.58 D for the one- and two-ring treatment groups, respectively)
- ○ regression of 0.1 D for the one-ring group and 0.2 D for the two-ring group (6 months to 2 years)
- • Vinciguerra et al, 1998 (effects of two different three-ring treatment patterns)
- ○ one session on 16 eyes of eight patients with a mean preoperative subjective cycloplegic refraction (SCR) of +4.90 ± 1.17 D
- • three eight-spot rings at ring diameters of 6, 7, or 8 mm
- ○ 10 pulses at a pulse energy of 240 mJ
- ○ treatment of one eye of each patient with a "radial" pattern (the spots of the three

rings aligned on the eight semimeridians)
- ○ treatment of the fellow eye with a "staggered" pattern (the spots of the contiguous rings offset 22.5 degrees from each other)
- ○ postoperative mean SCR of +2.75 ± 1.6 D in eyes treated with the radial pattern and +3.40 ± 1.6 D in eyes treated with the staggered pattern
- ○ mean change in SCR of 2.15 D and 1.50 D, respectively
- ○ mean improvement in UCVA of five lines in the radial eyes and four lines in the staggered eyes
- ○ earlier return of mean BCVA to preoperative levels in the radial group
- ○ one-year improvement of BCVA by one line in the radial eyes but no lines in staggered eyes
- ○ larger and more uniform corrected zones in the radial group [indicated by Scheimpflug photography and computerized videokeratography (CVK)]
- ○ because of this study all subsequent Ho:YAG LTK trials conducted using the radial pattern with either two or three rings

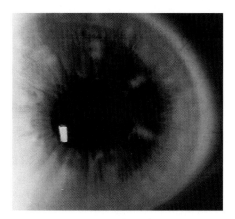

Figure 10–3 Slit-lamp photograph of patient treated with noncontact Ho:YAG LTK using two radially aligned rings.

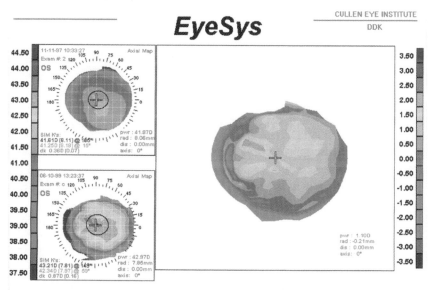

© 1990-1997 EyeSys Technologies Version 4.0

Figure 10–4 Preoperative CVK map (*upper left*), CVK map 17 months following noncontact Ho:YAG LTK (*lower left*), and a difference map (*right*).

- Koch et al[‡] (the FDA-monitored phase III studies of noncontact Ho:YAG LTK)
  - 648 hyperopic eyes (+0.75 to +2.50 D)
  - enrollment criteria as noted for prior studies (see above)

[‡]Presented at the American Society of Cataract and Refractive Surgery Symposium on Cataract, Intraocular Lens, and Refractive Surgery: April 1999; Seattle.

  - two concentric eight-spot rings at diameters of 6 to 7 mm
  - seven pulses per spot
  - pulse energies ranging from 226 to 256 mJ (Fig. 10–3)
  - reduction in hyperopia of 0.5 D or more in 92% of eyes [1.5–2.5 D in 39% of eyes (Fig. 10–4)]
  - loss of effect of 0.4 D from 6 to 12 months

- change in stability of less than 1 D in 95% of eyes by 6 months (FDA criterion is <1 D change in 95% of eyes at 3-month intervals)
- good predictability (65% of eyes within ±5 D of attempted correction and 88% of eyes within ±1.0 D of attempted)
- UCVA of ≥ 20/40 achieved in 86% of eyes and UCVA of ≥20/25 achieved in 57% of eyes
- reduction of full-time dependency on spectacles (from 79% to 13% in patients with hyperopia to +1.99 D and from 91 to 13% in patients with hyperopia of 2.0–2.5 D)
- loss of more than two lines of BCVA at 6 months in one patient (because of a cataract that was presumed to be unrelated to the treatment)
- indication of procedure as extremely safe and effective for treatment of low hyperopia (exceeded all FDA criteria by 6 months postoperatively)
- Acer et al[§]
  - 16 spots per ring with two rings at 6 and 7 mm (for treatment of hyperopia of 2.75–4.0 D)
  - mean corrections at 6 months slightly greater than 3 D
  - no reports of any sight-threatening complications
- Pop, 1998
  - noncontact Ho:YAG LTK in treating hyperopia following PRK for overcorrection of myopia after PRK
  - 36 eyes (33 patients) that underwent noncontact Ho:YAG LTK
  - no need for further retreatments for two-thirds of retreated eyes at 12 months after Ho:YAG LTK for an initial PRK

[§] Presented at the American Society of Cataract and Refractive Surgery Symposium on Cataract, Intraocular Lens, and Refractive Surgery: April 1999; Seattle.

- Ismail et al, 1998 (the efficacy and safety of noncontact Ho:YAG LTK)
  - 11 patients (13 eyes) with hyperopia induced by LASIK
  - eight pulses per spot
  - two staggered rings of eight spots at 6.0 and 7.0 mm
  - energy levels from 215 to 245 mJ
  - mean follow-up of 18 months
  - mean spherical equivalent of +4.60 D preoperatively, −0.5 D at 3 months, +0.48 D at 17 months, and +0.76 D at 18 months postoperatively
  - conclusion that Ho:YAG LTK is safe and effective for correcting LASIK-induced hyperopia (perhaps because of reduced corneal thickness and/or the presence of a circular incision in Bowman's membrane)

Complications
Sight-Threatening
- irregular astigmatism
  - In Summit FDA trials, 9% of patients lost at least two lines of BCVA in one year, which resolved over time.
  - U.S. and international studies performed with the Sunrise Corneal Shaping System have reported no treatment-induced loss of more than two lines of BCVA.
- visual aberrations (e.g., glare, loss of contrast sensitivity, decreased night vision)
  - In the Sunrise series, patients had no mean loss of contrast sensitivity, no loss of glare acuity, and did not complain of decreased night vision.
- visually significant corneal scarring
  - By 3 to 5 years postoperatively, treatment sites are not visible to the naked eye and are barely perceptible even by slit-lamp biomicroscopy.
  - Visual symptomatology because of the presence of the spots has not been reported.
- endothelial cell loss

- Patients in the Sunrise and Summit studies had no mean endothelial cell loss.
- infection (theoretically possible but no reports exist)

Non–Sight-Threatening

- undercorrection (caused by inadequate initial treatment or regression of effect)
  - The high incidence of regression led to abandonment of the Summit trials.
  - Efficacy is limited to adults older than 40 years who have hyperopia to 2.5 D (potentially extended to 4.0 D).
- overcorrection
  - Required in the first 3 to 6 months to compensate for early regression.
  - Long-term overcorrection is uncommon.
- increased astigmatism
  - In the phase III Sunrise study, induced manifest refractive cylinder of more than 2.00 D occurred in only 0.9% of eyes, which is well below the FDA threshold of 5%.
- RCEs
  - Theoretically possible as a result of epithelial injury, but none have been reported.

FUTURE DIRECTIONS

Despite an experimental history of more than 100 years, Ho:YAG LTK is in its clinical infancy. Clinical studies are in progress in the United States to assess the role of noncontact Ho:YAG LTK in treating presbyopia by inducing myopia in an emmetropic eye. Work is underway to develop treatment patterns that can be used for correcting astigmatism.

Sunrise has developed a new noncontact laser, the Hyperion, to replace the Corneal Shaping System (Fig. 10–5); this new device has multiple advantages, including eye tracking, automatic delivery of the second ring without refocusing, and

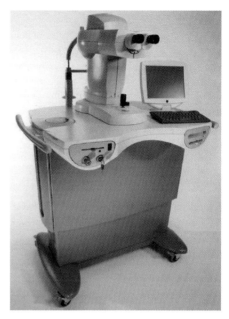

Figure 10–5 The Hyperion laser, which is the new noncontact Ho:YAG laser manufactured by Sunrise.

extraordinary programmability for spot placement and energy level.

A continuous-wave diode laser that emits energy at 1.885 μm (Rodenstock, Inc.) is now available in Europe and under clinical investigation for the treatment of hyperopia and hyperopic astigmatism. Finally, a nonlaser technology, radiofrequency thermal keratoplasty, is in the early stages of FDA study for treatment of low hyperopia.

As we better understand the response of the cornea to thermal change, devices, and treatment, we should expect improved parameters to further enhance the magnitude and stability of refractive change that can be produced by Ho:YAG LTK. We believe that Ho:YAG LTK is on the verge of becoming an integral part of the refractive surgical armamentarium.

Suggested Readings

Bende T, Jean B, Oltrup T. Laser thermal keratoplasty using a continuous wave diode laser. *J Refract Surg.* 1999;15:154–158.

Cavanaugh TB, Durrie DS. Holmium YAG laser thermokeratoplasty: synopsis of clinical experience. *Semin Ophthalmol.* 1994;9: 110–116.

Durrie DS, Schumer J, Cavanaugh TB. Holmium laser thermokeratoplasty for hyperopia. *J Refract Corneal Surg.* 1994;10:S277–S280.

Feldman ST, Ellis W, Frucht-Pery J, Chayet A, Brown SI. Regression of effect following radial thermokeratoplasty in humans. *J Refract Corneal Surg.* 1989;5:288–291.

Gasset AR, Kaufman HE. Thermokeratoplasty in the treatment of keratoconus. *Am J Ophthalmol.* 1975;79:226–232.

Ismail MM, Alió JL, Pérez-Sntonja JJ. Noncontact thermal keratoplasty to correct hyperopia induced by laser in situ keratomileusis. *J Refract Surg.* 1998;24:1191–1194.

Ismail MM, Pérez-Sntonja JJ, Alió JL. Laser thermal keratoplasty after lamellar corneal cutting. *J Refract Surg.* 1999;25:212–215.

Koch DD, Abarca A, Villarreal R, et al. Hyperopia correction by noncontact holmium: YAG laser thermal keratoplasty: clinical study with 2-year follow-up. *Ophthalmology.* 1996; 103:731–740.

Koch DD, Kohnen T, McDonnell PJ, Menefee RF, Berry MJ. Hyperopia correction by noncontact holmium:YAG laser thermal keratoplasty: U.S. phase IIa clinical study with 2-year follow-up. *Ophthalmology.* 1997;104: 1938–1947.

McDonnell PJ, Garbus J, Romero N, Rao A, Schanzlin DJ. Electrosurgical keratoplasty: clinicopathologic correlation. *Arch Ophthalmol.* 1988;106:235–238.

Moriera H, Campus M, Sawusch MR, McDonnell JM, Sand B, McDonnell PJ.

Holmium laser keratoplasty. *Ophthalmology.* 1993;100:752–761.

Neumann AC, Fyodorov S, Sanders DR. Radial thermokeratoplasty for the correction of hyperopia. *J Refract Corneal Surg.* 1990;6:404–412.

Peyman GA, Larson B, Raichand M, Andrews AH. Modification of rabbit corneal curvature with the use of carbon dioxide laser burns. *Ophthalmic Surg.* 1980;11:325–329.

Pop M. Laser thermal keratoplasty for the treatment of photorefractive keratectomy overcorrections: a 1-year follow-up. *Ophthalmology.* 1998;105:926–931.

Rowsey JJ, Doss JD. Preliminary report of Los Alamos keratoplasty techniques. *Ophthalmology.* 1981;88:755–760.

Seiler T. Ho:YAG laser thermokeratoplasty for hyperopia. *Ophthalmol Clinics North Am.* 1992; 5:773–780.

Seiler T, Matallana M, Bende T. Laser thermokeratoplasty by means of a pulsed holmium:YAG laser for hyperopic correction. *J Refract Corneal Surg.* 1990;6:335–339.

Stringer H, Parr J. Shrinkage temperature of eye collagen. *Nature.* 1964;204:1307.

Thompson VM. Holmium:YAG laser thermokeratoplasty for correction of astigmatism. *J Refract Corneal Surg.* 1994;10:S293.

Vinciguerra P, Azzolini M, Radice P, Epstein D, Kohnen T, Koch DD. Comparison of radial and staggered treatment patterns for the correction of hyperopia in noncontact holmium:YAG laser thermal keratoplasty. *J Cataract Refract Surg.* 1998;24:21–30.

Yanoff M. Holium laser hyperopia thermokeratoplasty update. *Eur J Implant Refract Surg.* 1995;7:89–91.

Zhou Z, Ren QS, Simon G, Parel JM. Thermal modeling of laser photothermo-keratoplasty (LPTK). *SPIE Proc.* 1992;1644:61–71.

CHAPTER 11

Laser In Situ Keratomileusis

Louis E. Probst and John F. Doane

CHAPTER CONTENTS

Lamellar corneal surgery for the correction of refractive errors has been evolving for 50 years since Professor Jose I. Barraquer of Bogota, Colombia, invented the field in 1948. Many of his concepts continue to guide this particular field of ophthalmic surgery, and much of today's instrumentation originated from his ideas.

Refractive lamellar corneal surgery attempts to remove, add, or modify the corneal stroma to alter the tear film/anterior corneal interface radius of curvature. For the treatment of myopia, tissue may be removed centrally [i.e., via myopic laser in situ keratomileusis (LASIK)] or added peripherally [i.e., by insertion of an intracorneal ring (ICR)] to induce central corneal flattening and reduction of myopia. For hyperopia, tissue may be added centrally (i.e., through keratophakia), subtracted peripherally (i.e., via hyperopic LASIK), or affected by a deep keratectomy with controlled ectasia [i.e., automated lamellar keratoplasty (ALK) for hyperopia], which may be performed to induce central corneal steepening with a reduction of

spherical plus refractive power. Treatment of astigmatism is accomplished by flattening the steep axis or steepening the flat axis (to remove tissue) to make the overall cornea spherical.

THE EVOLUTION OF LAMELLAR REFRACTIVE SURGERY

The surgical techniques used in lamellar refractive surgery have evolved toward increased simplicity and greater patient safety. The end results have been improvement in refractive results and wider acceptance of the procedures by surgeons. Several distinct techniques for performing lamellar surgery exist today.

General Advantages
- ability to treat a larger range of refractive errors
- shorter visual rehabilitation time
- minimal postoperative discomfort
- reduced healing response compared with photorefractive keratectomy (PRK)

- relative ease of enhancement compared with PRK

General Disadvantages
- need for advanced technical expertise
- large ongoing capital expenditures
- potential for serious intraoperative complications (see pp. 121–122)

Instrumentation
- microkeratome (Figs. 11–1 and 11–2)
  - functions like a carpenter's plane to perform a planar (no refractive power) resection of anterior cornea tissue
  - contains an oscillating blade that incises the tissue at an even depth [if intraocular pressure (IOP) is constant and the microkeratome moves across the cornea at a constant velocity]

Freeze Keratomileusis
The term "keratomileusis" derives from the Greek roots *keras* (horn-like: cornea) and *mileusis* (carving). In 1949, Barraquer developed freeze keratomileusis, which alters the cornea's refractive power by shaping the cornea itself. However, because of its many disadvantages, freeze myopic keratomileusis is no longer performed.

Disadvantages
- steep learning curve for performing the keratectomy and using the cryolathe

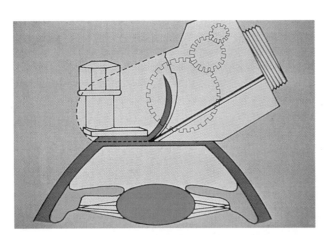

Figure 11–1 Keratome creating a lamellar dissection by applanating the cornea like a carpenter's plane. (Courtesy of Stephen G. Slade, M.D.)

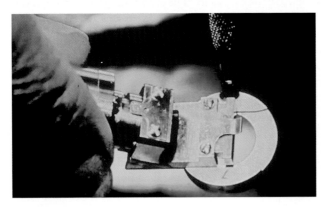

Figure 11–2 Manual Barraquer microkeratome and suction ring. (Courtesy of Stephen G. Slade, M.D.)

- dependence on the constant velocity of the manual microkeratome to maintain the thickness and evenness of the keratectomy
- possibility of irregular astigmatism and a loss of best-corrected visual acuity (BCVA) from any keratectomy irregularity
- difficulty mastering and maintaining skill with the cryolathe
- lack of ability to transfer skills to many other procedures
- availability of better options (e.g., LASIK)
- difficulty placing antitorque sutures

Indications and Inclusion Criteria
- myopia (≤ -15 to -18 D)
- hyperopia ($\leq +6$ D)
- not for treatment of astigmatism

Methods (Fig. 11–3)
- Harvest 300 µm of the corneal cap.
- Stain the corneal cap with Chiton-green stain.
- Invert the cap epithelial-side down on a freezing block.

- Sculpt the back (stromal side) surface with a cryolathe (Figs. 11–4 and 11–5).
- Reposition the cap on the stromal bed.
- Suture the cap in place.
- Remove sutures 2 to 3 weeks after complete epithelialization.

Keratomileusis In Situ for Myopia

Barraquer also conceived the process of raising a corneal cap and removing central tissue from the bed. Krwawicz and Pureskin described similar techniques as "central stromectomy." Because of several disadvantages and the frequency of certain complications, this technique is no longer practiced.

Disadvantages
- availability of a better option (i.e., LASIK)
- difficulty placing antitorque sutures

Indications and Inclusion Criteria
- myopia (≤ -18 D)
- not for treatment of astigmatism

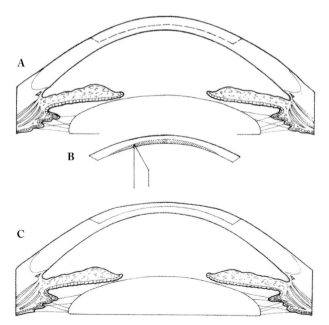

Figure 11–3 Freeze Myopic Keratomileusis. (A) 300-µm corneal cap created with microkeratome. (B) Central stroma from posterior aspect of cap removed with cryolathe. (C) Cap replaced and sutured in place with antitorque suture. Central cornea has been flattened to reduce myopia.

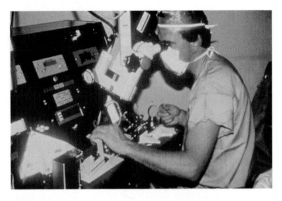

Figure 11–4 Surgical team member operating the cryolathe. (Courtesy of Stephen G. Slade, M.D.)

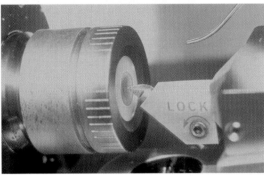

Figure 11–5 Cryolathing of a lamellar corneal disk. (Photo courtesy of Stephen G. Slade, M.D.)

Methods (Fig. 11–6)

- Create a free cap to gain access to the corneal stroma using a manual pass of the microkeratome.
- Remove a smaller-diameter disc of tissue with a second pass of the microkeratome across the stromal bed.
- Determine the size of the refractive correction with the thickness of the second "power cut."
- Replace the cap to reduce corneal curvature and myopia.
- Suture the cap in place using an anti-torque technique.

Complications

- infection
- irregular astigmatism (frequent)
- loss of cap
- lamellar complications (epithelial ingrowth and flap melting)

Keratophakia

Keratophakia means "corneal lens." Barraquer first developed the procedure keratophakia in the 1960s as a treatment for aphakia after intracapsular cataract extraction. With the advent of extracapsular and phacoemulsification cataract surgery techniques along with improved intraocular lens (IOL) technology, keratophakia has been relegated to a lesser role; surgical aphakia is no longer a prevalent problem. The future role of keratophakia or corneal inlay techniques in refractive surgery may involve the addition of synthetic tissue or lens material under a flap or placement of a transparent material of a different (or same) index of refraction from the corneal stroma in a stromal pocket to correct myopia, hyperopia, astigmatism, or presbyopia.

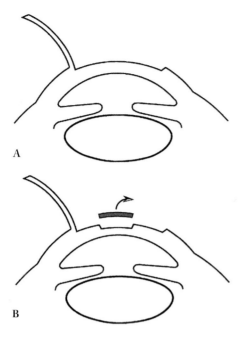

Figure 11-6 Keratomileusis in situ for myopia [manual or automated lamellar keratoplasty]. (A) Creation of corneal flap with first pass of a microkeratome.

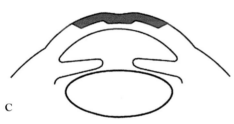

(B) Removal of central stromal tissue from bed (refractive cut) with the second pass of the microkeratome.

(C) Reposit flap. Central cornea has been flattened for treatment of myopia.

Indications and Inclusion Criteria
- hyperopia (typically ≤ ~6 D)
- aphakia (≤ 14 D)
- not for treatment of astigmatism

Methods (Fig. 11–7)
- Create a flap and/or cap.
- Place a disc of tissue underneath the flap and/or cap to increase the central corneal curvature.
- Typically, harvest the tissue to be added from donor corneal tissue using a microkeratome.
- Select a specific disc diameter and thickness of tissue based on the patient's refractive error.

Complications
- infection
- irregular astigmatism
- loss of cap
- lamellar complications (epithelial ingrowth and flap melting)
- decentration of lens inlay
- loss of BCVA

Barraquer-Krumeich-Swinger Nonfreeze Keratomileusis Technique
The goal of the Barraquer-Krumeich-Swinger (BKS) technique was the improvement of refractive results and the simplification of lamellar surgery. The procedure is no longer performed.

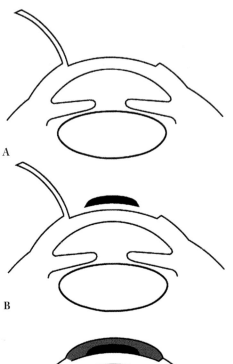

Figure 11–7 Keratophakia (homoplastic allograft or synthetic inlay). (A) Creation of flap or cap.

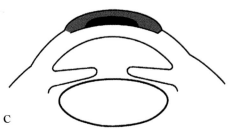

(B) Graft inlay positioned over central stromal bed.

(C) Flap or cap repositioned. Central corneal power increased effectively treating hyperopia or aphakia.

Advantages
- avoidance of adverse tissue effects (loss of fibroblasts) associated with freezing of the corneal cap
- preservation of the corneal epithelium with a more comfortable postoperative course of healing
- light processing of the tissue
- maintenance of the intact epithelium

Disadvantages
- availability of a better option (i.e., LASIK)

- technical difficulty performing refractive keratectomy
- difficulty placing antitorque sutures
- frequency of postoperative irregular astigmatism

Indications and Inclusion Criteria
- myopia (≤ -18 D)
- hyperopia ($\leq +6$ D)
- not for treatment of astigmatism

Methods (Figs. 11–8 and 11–9)
- See the initial methods for freeze keratomileusis.

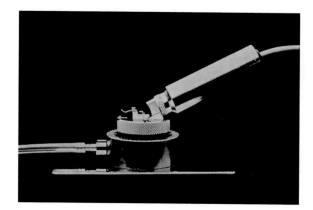

Figure 11–8 Barraquer-Krumeich-Swinger microkeratome and suction platform. (Courtesy of Stephen G. Slade, M.D.)

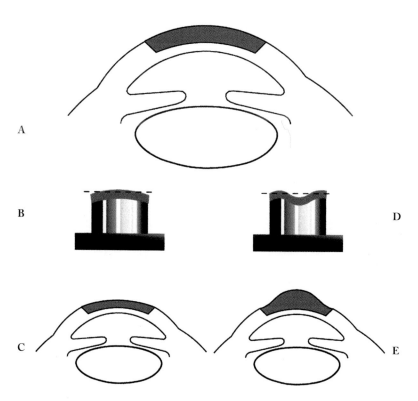

Figure 11–9 Barraquer-Krumeich-Swinger keratomileusis technique. (A) 300-μm cap created with microkeratome. (B) Cap placed epithelial-side down on suction dye. Stroma removed from central aspect of the posterior aspect cap with manual microkeratome. (C) Cap reposited with antitorque sutures. Central cornea flattened for treatment of myopia. (D) Cap placed epithelial-side down on suction dye. Tissue removed from paracentral stroma of posterior cap with manual microkeratome. (E) Cap reposited. Corneal curvature has been steepened for treatment of hyperopia.

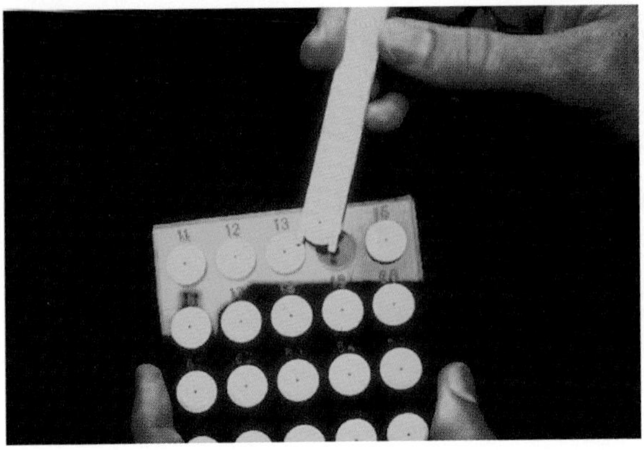

Figure 11–10 Barraquer-Krumeich-Swinger suction dyes. (Courtesy of Stephen G. Slade, M.D.)

- Harvest a 300-μm corneal cap using the BKS microkeratome.
- Place the cap epithelial-side down on one of several specific suction dyes.
- Choose the suction dye based on the planned diopter correction of myopia or hyperopia (Fig. 11–10).
- Make the refractive cut with the microkeratome.
- Suture the cap in place with the anti-torque technique.

Complications
- infection
- irregular astigmatism (frequent and major drawback)
- loss of cap
- lamellar complications (epithelial ingrowth and flap melting)

Epikeratophakia
The first "Americanized" version of a lamellar refractive surgery technique was epikeratophakia/epikeratoplasty as described by Kaufman and Werblin. What seemed to be a modernization of lamellar surgery ultimately was not a viable alternative.

Advantages
- automation of the difficult task of using the cryolathe

- provision of a high-quality, preprocessed refractive corneal lenticule from a centralized manufacturer that freezes and cryolathes specific corrective powers, lyophilizes the lenticule in a sterile bottle (Fig. 11–11), and then ships it to the surgeon.

Disadvantages
- variability of surgical results
- poor profitability for the manufacturer of the lenticules
- emergence of better alternative therapies (e.g., IOLs and laser refractive techniques)

Indications and Inclusion Criteria
- treatment of the following for children and adults
  - aphakia
  - myopia
  - hyperopia
  - keratoconus
  - keratoglobus
- not for treatment of astigmatism

Methods
- Reconstitute the lenticule with balanced salt solution (BSS).
- Suture the lenticule onto the eye after host-bed preparation (Fig. 11–12).

Complications
- those associated with re-epithelialization over the donor lenticule

REFRACTIVE SURGERY: A COLOR SYNOPSIS

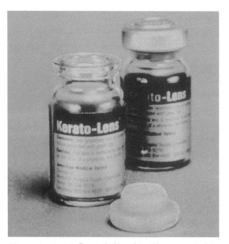

Figure 11–11 Lyophilized epikeratophakia lenticule in transport bottle labeled with refractive power.

∘ delayed healing
∘ interface epithelial ingrowth
∘ lenticule melting or necrosis
• infection

• irregular astigmatism
• loss of cap

Automated Keratomileusis In Situ

The next major advance in the field of lamellar refractive surgery was development of the motorized Ruiz microkeratome, which was invented by another Colombian surgeon and protégé of Barraquer, Dr. Luis Antonio Ruiz. ALK is no longer performed.

Advantages
• gears that advance the microkeratome across a geared track
• an adjustable-height suction ring (defined the technique now known as ALK; Fig. 11–13)
• a constant passage velocity
• a lamellar tissue disc of even thickness
• a smoother corneal stromal bed
• increased appeal for a larger number of surgeons who found manual microkeratomes difficult to master

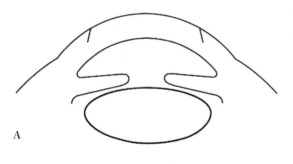

A

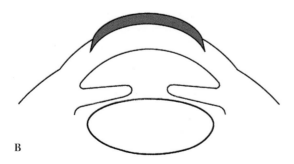

B

Figure 11–12 Epikeratophakia. (A) Preparation of the recipient bed by removing the epithelium and creating a 360-degree circumferential flange after epithelial removal.

(B) Prefabricated onlay lenticule is positioned under flange edge and sutured in place. Depending on the lenticule power, myopic, hyperopic, or aphakic refractive errors may be treated.

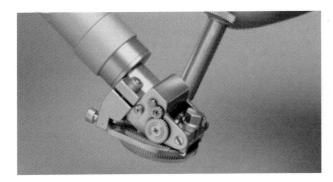

Figure 11–13 Automated geared microkeratome and geared-track of suction ring.

Disadvantages
- availability of a better option (i.e., LASIK)
- abandonment of the hyperopic technique because of concern about progressive ectasia
- technical demands of procedure

Indications and Inclusion Criteria
- myopia (≤ -20 D)
- hyperopia ($\leq +6$ D)
- not for treatment of astigmatism

Methods
- Perform ALK in an outpatient setting with topical anesthesia (oral sedation is optional).
- Irrigate the conjunctival cul-de-sacs to remove debris and eyelid glandular secretions.
- Clean eyelids in the standard manner with povidone-iodine solution (Betadine).
- Drape the eyelids.
  - creates a clear path for microkeratome passage
  - removes the lashes and extraneous periocular tissue from the surgical field
- Instruct the patient to look at the microscope light.
- With an inked marker, delineate the optical center, a pararadial line for orientation of the flap, and a 9-mm optical-zone (OZ) circle to center the circular suction ring (Fig. 11–14).
- Place a spacer device (or depth plate) in the microkeratome to determine the thickness of the cut. (The first keratectomy in ALK typically utilizes a 160-μm depth plate.)

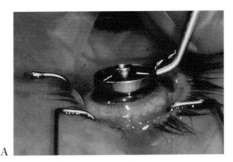
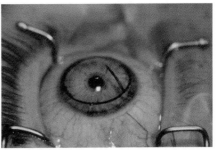

A   B

Figure 11–14 (A and B) A Ruiz marker is impregnated with ink and used to make a pararadial mark for orientation of the flap and 9-mm OZ for proper placement of the suction ring. (Courtesy of Stephen G. Slade, M.D.)

- Place an adjustable suction ring on the eye and engage the suction to do the following.
  - fixate the globe
  - provide a geared path for the microkeratome
  - raise the IOP to allow presentation of adequate corneal tissue (enables a smooth keratectomy of even thickness)
- Create a hinge in the corneal flap with a stopper device.
- Just prior to passage of the microkeratome, use a hand-held Barraquer tonometer to check the IOP to ensure that it is greater than 65 mmHg.
- Remove the suction ring after the first cut, which has a planned diameter of 7.5 to 8.0 mm.
- Reset the adjustable suction ring to resect a 4.2-mm-diameter piece of stromal tissue.
- Place a second depth plate, which corresponds to the planned myopic correction.
- Replace the suction ring and make a second cut (the "power cut") after checking the diameter and the IOP.
- Replace the flap and position it without sutures.

- Protect the patient's eye with a clear, plastic orbital shield (Fig. 11–15) and discharge the patient with broad-spectrum topical antibiotics
- Examine the eye the next day.

Complications
- infection
- irregular astigmatism
- loss of cap
- lamellar complications (epithelial ingrowth and flap melting)
- significant loss of BCVA (5–10% in some studies)

LASER IN SITU KERATOMILEUSIS

The postoperative complications of central corneal haze, regression of effect, and diminished efficacy for myopia over −6 D with excimer laser PRK and the predictable shortcomings of ALK led to the development of LASIK. Researchers substituted lasers for the keratome in the refractive correction step of the myopic ALK procedure and LASIK was born. Some researchers postulated that the submicron ablation

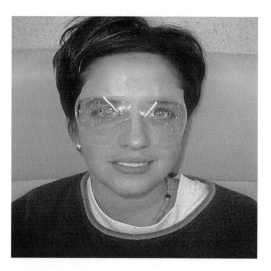

Figure 11–15 A plastic orbital shield is used to protect the globe from direct physical contact for three to four nights while asleep.

precision of the excimer laser allows for much more predictable refractive results that do not depend as heavily on individual patient healing responses, as had been noted with PRK.

Preoperative Considerations

Advantages
- incredible precision of tissue removal
- minimal postoperative discomfort
- early recovery of visual function
- immediate return to preoperative lifestyle
- lack of topical steroid usage
- lack of concern for undesirable healing phenomena (e.g., haze formation)
- a short postoperative antibiotic regimen
- less-intensive follow-up than that for PRK
- increased range of efficacy for myopia, hyperopia, and astigmatism (compared with PRK)

Indications and Inclusion Criteria*
- myopia (0.5–15.0 D)
- hyperopia (0.5–6.0 D)
- regular astigmatism (≤ 8 D)
- patient at least 18 years of age (as for refractive surgery in general)[†]
- refractive stability (≥ 12 months)
- clarity of the crystalline lens
- education about the alternative refractive surgical procedures (e.g., radial keratotomy, PRK, ICR segments, clear lens extraction, or phakic IOL placement)

---

*These ranges are not absolute; many surgeons have successfully treated patients with myopia, hyperopia, or astigmatism beyond these ranges. Other surgeons may work at lower ranges based on their personal experience with the procedure.
[†]The use of LASIK for equalization of refractive error between eyes of pediatric patients has been done outside the United States but remains controversial.

- evaluation of patient expectations
- completion of informed consent form

Preoperative Patient Evaluation
- visual acuity testing
- refraction
  - manifest refraction (duochrome test and fogging techniques)
  - cycloplegic refraction (to check excessive accommodation during manifest examination)
  - comparison of refraction with prior spectacle corrections to assess the stability of refraction
  - discontinuation of soft contact lens wear at least 3 days to preferably 2 weeks prior to examination
  - discontinuation of rigid gas-permeable (RGP) lens wear at least 3 weeks before first of at least two examinations performed 3 days apart
  - at least 0.25 D difference in refraction (validates stability)
- evaluation of central corneal thickness using pachymetry (assesses safe limits of corneal stromal removal with laser ablation by measuring flap thickness, depth of ablation, and residual thickness of the stromal bed after ablation)
  - A thin flap more likely leads to irregular astigmatism and lost lines of BCVA.
  - A flap at least 160 μm thick minimizes induced irregular astigmatism.
  - A thin stromal bed (<250 μm) may increase the likelihood of central ectasia with long-term unstable refractive status.
  - For example, central pachymetry (560 μm) − flap thickness (160 μm) = preablation stromal bed (400 μm) so in this case ablate no more that 200 μm of stromal bed.
  - Based on the Munnerlynn formula (ablation depth = optical zone^2 × diopters treated/3), no more than 15 D

of myopia could be treated if using a 6-mm OZ.

- If preoperative central corneal thickness is thinner and ablation still leaves a 200-μm-thick stromal bed, less refractive error may be treated safely.
- Multizone ablations can correct larger amounts of refractive error because less tissue is removed than with single-zone ablations (overall OZ is smaller and night vision may be compromised).
- computerized videokeratography
- slit-lamp examination
- retinal evaluation
- eye-dominance testing
- evaluation for monovision (when appropriate) (see p. 66)
- evaluation for astigmatism
  - refraction
  - keratometry
  - videokeratography
- formulation of nomogram
  - Lasers come with algorithms for treating a specific refractive error.
  - Surgical technique, ideal room conditions (humidity, 30–50%; temperature, 18–24°C; filtration of low air particulate matter), and laser components (quality of optics, gas mixture) directly impact the refractive result and are laser algorithm–independent but addressed by the individual surgeon nomogram.
  - Clearly follow a methodical calculation scheme when determining what data to enter into the laser for each eye to be treated.
  - A worksheet in the patient's chart prevents calculation mishaps (Table 11–1).

Absolute Contraindications
- unstable refraction
- keratoconus
- irregular astigmatism
- inadequate corneal thickness
- active corneal or ocular disease

Relative Contraindications
- thin corneas
- active collagen vascular disease
- systemic vasculitis
- low endothelial cell counts (<500–1500 cells/mm^2)
- anterior basement dystrophy
- history of recurrent erosions (an epithelial defect can occur during the keratectomy and lead to poor flap adhesion with subsequent epithelial ingrowth and flap melting; surgeon experience helps to avoid epithelial ingrowth)
- pregnancy or lactation (may be considered if stable through prior pregnancies and have no refractive change from current eyewear; J.F.D. has treated several pregnant and lactating women after careful consent and thorough evaluation of their previous refraction history)
- history of herpes simplex or herpes zoster keratitis (use prophylactic oral

TABLE 11–1
Sample Items on Worksheet for LASIK Nomogram

Line 1 (preoperative refraction)	−6.0 D sphere
Line 2 (postoperative target)	plano
Line 3 (line 1–line 2)	−6.0 D sphere
Line 4 (% reduction or addition; presume 90% of sphere)	−5.4 D sphere
Line 5 (treatment entered into laser)	−5.4 D sphere

and/or topical antiviral agents periopera- tively because of risk for stromal melt- ing; proceed very carefully with these patients)
• patients with monocular vision

Surgical Considerations

At least two different techniques have been used for laser myopic keratomileusis: LASIK and the Buratto technique. LASIK is now the predominant technique because the sutureless hinged flap is sig- nificantly easier to deal with compared with correctly orientating a free cap onto the stromal bed (Figs. 11–16 and 11–17). The Buratto technique is analogous to freeze myopic keratomileusis (MKM) except for substitution of the excimer laser

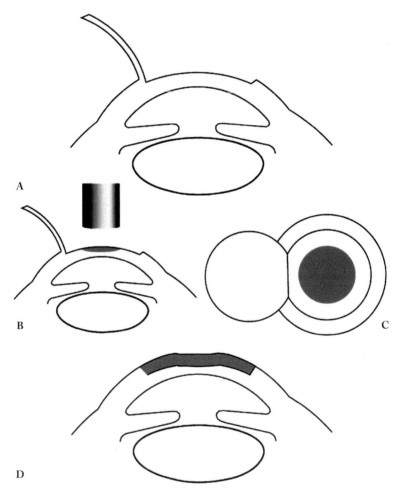

Figure 11–16 Laser in situ keratomileusis for myopia. (A) Creation of flap. (B) Laser ablation of stromal bed and tissue removal (shaded area). (C) Shaded area represents zone of tissue removal (top view). (D) Flap replaced and central cornea flattened.

for the cryolathe in the refractive step of the procedure.

- LASIK
  - Create a hinged flap.
  - Remove corneal stroma from the bed with the laser.

- Treat sphere and cylinder depending on the capabilities of the laser (Figs. 11–18 to 11–20).
- The Buratto technique
  - Remove a thick disc of tissue (300–350 μm) completely from the eye.

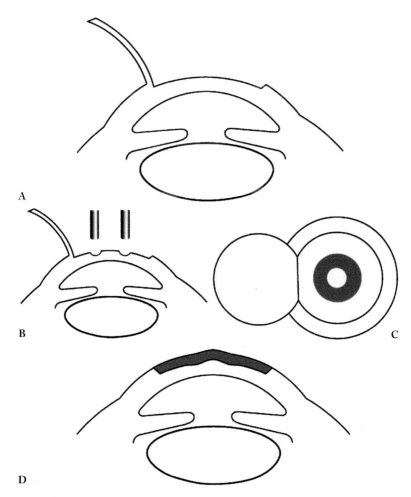

Figure 11–17 Laser in situ keratomileusis for hyperopia. (A) Creation of flap. (B) Laser ablation of stromal bed and paracentral tissue removal (shaded area). (C) Shaded area represents zone of tissue removal (top view). (D) Flap replaced and central cornea steepened.

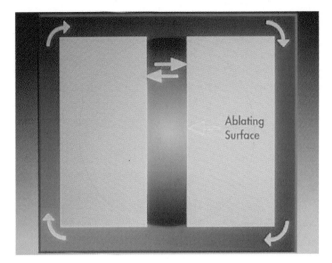

Figure 11–18 VISX Star astigmatic correction. Parallel blades allow preferential ablation parallel to the minus cylinder axis or the flat corneal meridian, which in effect flattens the steep corneal axis.

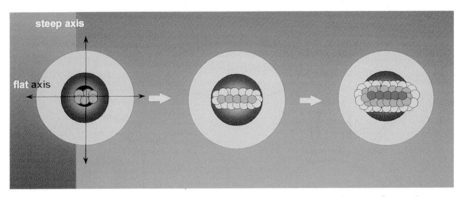

Figure 11–19 Schematic of minus cylinder ablation with scanning spot laser to flatten the steep corneal meridian.

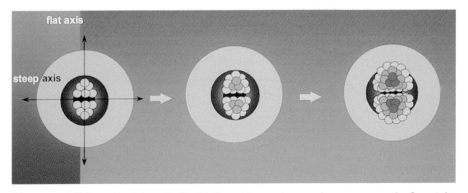

Figure 11–20 Schematic of plus cylinder ablation with scanning spot laser to steepen the flat axis by removing tissue paracentrally parallel to the minus cylinder axis or the flat axis on keratometry.

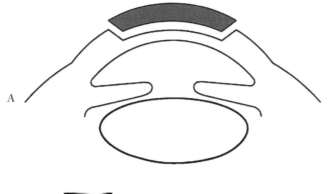

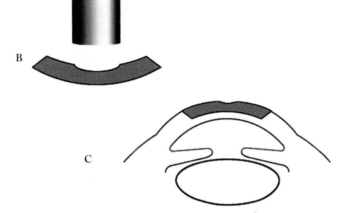

Figure 11–21 Buratto style laser keratomileusis. (A) Creation of thick (300-μm) "free" cap. (B) Inversion of cap and laser used to remove central cap stroma (shaded area). (C) Reposition of cap in keratectomy bed. Central cornea has been flattened to treat myopia.

○ Place the disc beneath the laser stroma side up and ablate with the excimer laser (Fig. 11–21).
○ Replace the disc of tissue on the eye.

Instrument Setup and Surgical Team Mentality
• Select a laser depending on desired ablation depth.
  ○ most lasers: 12 to 15 μm/D (in 6-mm single zone algorithms)
  ○ VISX Star (VISX, Inc., Santa Clara, CA): 15 μm/SE diopter (6-mm single-zone algorithm)

○ VISX Smoothscan: 12 μm/SE diopter (6-mm single-zone algorithm)
• Consider the amount of residual stroma.
  ○ 160-μm plate leaves a 150 ± 20 μm flap
  ○ 200 to 250 μm should be left in stromal bed (U.S. Federal Department of Agriculture now recommends 250 μm)
  ○ ideal total corneal thickness = 150 + 250 μm
• Select a keratome based on keratometry values (Ks).
  ○ Ks < 42.0 D [200-μm plate with the Automated Corneal Shaper (ACS) or Hansatome (Bausch & Lomb, Rochester, NY)]

- $Ks = 42–46$ D (160–180 μm plate with ACS or Hansatome)
- $Ks > 46$ D (160-μm plate or Hansatome)
- Properly clean, assemble, and test the microkeratome.
- Calibrate and set up the laser.
  - Check fluence (proper energy setting in mJ/cm^2).
  - Check beam homogeneity (evenness of energy distribution across surface area).
- Each team member is responsible for every aspect of the procedure and should complete multiple checks as the procedure progresses.
- Ensure appropriate humidity, temperature, and air purification in the laser room at all times to preserve laser optics and establish standardized treatment conditions.

Patient Preparation
- Administer 5 to 10 mg of diazepam orally approximately 45 min prior to the procedure.
- Do *not* use a preoperative miotic.
- Irrigate the conjunctival fornices with eyewash to remove any meibomian secretions or tear-film debris.
- Clean eyelids with Betadine.
- Position the patient under the laser in the supine position with the frontal surface of the cornea perpendicular to the laser-beam aperture.
- Instill 1 to 2 drops of a mild topical anesthetic (e.g., proparacaine).
- Dry the eyelashes with a gauze sponge and place a fenestrated drape over eyelashes to keep them and redundant periocular tissues out of the surgical field.
- Insert a wire-locking eyelid speculum (allows adequate exposure).

The Keratectomy
- Open the speculum another 1 to 2 mm after waiting 1 min after initial insertion.

- Mark the corneal epithelium with a lamellar corneal surgery marker (useful for proper positioning of a free cap; see Fig. 11–14).
- Place the LASIK pneumatic suction ring onto the eye to provide globe fixation, elevation of IOP to create an even-thickness keratectomy, and a track for the advancement of the microkeratome.
- Press down suction ring.
- After activating the vacuum to the pneumatic suction ring, directly check the IOP using a Barraquer tonometer, pneumotonometer, or digital palpation.
- Ensure that the path of the microkeratome is clear.
- Pull down the lower lid with the Hansatome.
- After obtaining sufficient IOP, lubricate the corneal surface with BSS or proparicaine to minimize epithelium disruption while making a pass with the microkeratome.
- Load the microkeratome into the dovetailed groove on the suction ring and then advance and reverse it.
- Double depress at the end of the cut to ensure completion.
- Discontinue vacuuming and remove the LASIK suction ring or hold the eye with the suction ring while suction is off during the laser ablation.

Laser Ablation
- Before lifting the flap, the surgeon and staff should confirm proper laser settings and position the patient's head so that the corneal surface is perpendicular to the ablation beam.
- Lift the flap and fold it out of the ablation field.
- Center the ablation over the entrance pupil (critical for hyperopes).
  - Monitor the centration cautiously.
  - If significant movement occurs, stop the ablation, reorient the patient (center eye

by raising patient's chin and turn head nasally for small palpebral apertures), and proceed when the centration is aligned.

- Use an eye tracker or eye fixation for nystagmus, mobile eyes, or hyperopic eyes.
- Turn down the microscope light.
- Wipe dry any ablation fluid that accumulates on the corneal surface with a single pass of a nonfragmenting cellulose sponge or blunt spatula.
- As the ablation proceeds to the largest-diameter treatment zones, cover the hinge with a blunt instrument, if necessary, to prevent ablation of the back surface of the corneal flap.
- If treating concurrent astigmatism, ensure the appropriate axis of treatment by marking a reference point on the patient's limbus prior to initiating the treatment session.
- If significant cyclotorsion occurs when placing the patient in the supine position, adjust the axis that is programmed into the laser.
- Correct astigmatism by differentially removing tissue in the frontal plane of the cornea in one of the two major meridians (flatten the steep axis, steepen the flat axis, or perform crossed-cylinder ablation).
  - minus cylinder format [Flatten the steep axis by using large-area ablation lasers with closing blades (see Fig. 11–18), masking systems, or flying-spot lasers by passing the spot parallel to the minus cylinder axis or flat axis on keratometry (see Fig. 11–19). It is best used for myopic astigmatism because it minimizes tissue removal.]
  - plus cylinder format [Steepen the flat axis best with scanning-spot lasers by removing tissue paracentrally parallel to the minus cylinder axis or flatter axis on keratometry (see Fig. 11–20). It is best used for hyperopic astigmatism because it minimizes tissue removal.]
  - crossed cylinder format [Use this method for mixed astigmatism in which each major meridian receives a combination of steepening or flattening, respectively (Fig. 11–22).]

Repositioning the Flap

- Gently float the flap into the stromal bed at the completion of the laser ablation.
- Place a small-gauge cannula underneath the flap and irrigate for 5 to 10 sec with BSS in a closed system to clear any remaining debris from the interface (increased irrigation time decreases adhesion of the flap and leads to flap edema with greater flap-edge gape; Fig. 11–23).
- Inspect the flap to ensure proper positioning by verifying that an equal gutter (keratectomy edge) distance is present throughout the circumference (Fig. 11–24).
- Check corneal alignment marks.
- Allow the interface to dry for several minutes.
  - During the drying phase we recommend that you administer a microdrop of BSS over the central corneal epithelium to maintain its integrity.
- Test flap adhesion by performing a striae test.
  - Depress the peripheral cornea with closed blunt-tipped forceps.
  - When striae pass well into the flap 360 degrees, you have achieved appropriate adhesion.
- Remove the speculum and drape.
- Reexamine the eye to ensure that the flap is properly positioned.
- Instill a topical broad spectrum antibiotic (Ciloxan; Alcon) and nonsteroidal anti-inflammatory medication drop (Voltaren; CibaVision).
- Place a shield over the orbit but do not apply a pressure patch.

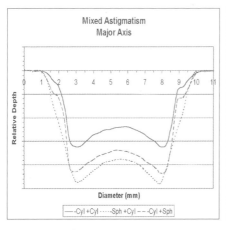
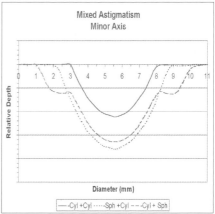

Figure 11–22 Crossed-cylinder ablation versus plus and minus cylinder ablation profiles for the treatment of mixed astigmatism. Note less depth is required to achieve identical refractive correction in both the major and minor axes for crossed-cylinder profile (red curve) compared with minus cylinder profile (green) and plus cylinder profile (blue).

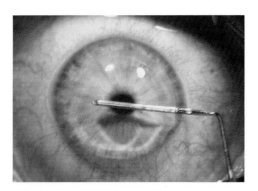

Figure 11–23 Doane-Slade superior hinge irrigating cannula under closed flap. Note the "closed system" irrigation of BSS to clear the interface of debris.

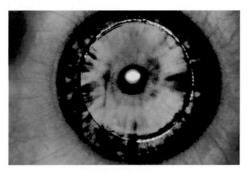

Figure 11–24 The reposited flap should be inspected for equal gutter/keratectomy edge distance throughout its circumference. (Courtesy of Stephen G. Slade, M.D.)

Postoperative Considerations

Typical postoperative care of a LASIK patient is relatively simple.

Results
- generally no pain
- foreign body sensation, light sensitivity, and tearing (typically present for the first few hours after surgery)
- uncorrected visual acuity (UCVA) of 20/40 or better in the low and moderate myopia treatment ranges
- a clear cornea with intact epithelium on slit-lamp examination
- proper flap apposition (check)
- stromal edema or interface debris (document)

Patient Management
- Prescribe topical prophylactic antibiotics 4 times a day for the first week.
- Prescribe topical corticosteroids for the first 4 to 7 days postoperatively.
- Topical preservative-free lubricating drops may help select patients (as needed) for several weeks after surgery.
- Use an orbital shield to protect the globe from direct pressure during the first 3 to 4 nights.

- Systemic analgesics are rarely necessary.
- Instruct the patient to resume normal activities after the 1 day postoperative examination (if results are normal), but caution the patient to avoid rubbing the cornea and participating in contact sports without proper eye protection.
- Instruct the patient to avoid exposure to potentially contaminated moisture sources such as hot tubs, pools, and fresh-water lakes for at least 2 weeks.
- Tell the patient that full visual recovery may take several weeks or more and may be delayed if significant irregular astigmatism exists.

FLAP COMPLICATIONS Flaps may be too short, too thin, irregular, or free (free cap) (Fig. 11–25 to 11–27). An alteration of the various forces during the LASIK procedure (Table 11–2) may explain their occurrence.

Prevention
- Properly assemble and prepare the microkeratome.
- Training the surgeon and staff is the cornerstone for achieving reproducible high-quality lamellar incisions.

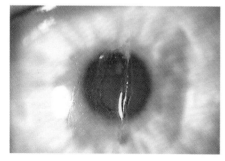

Figure 11–25 A centrally perforated flap immediately after LASIK.

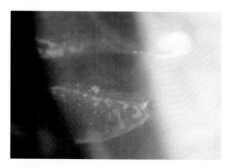

Figure 11–26 A horizontal linear flap defect because of a defective blade 4 months after LASIK.

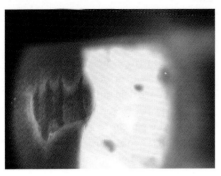

Figure 11–27 A central flap perforation with skip marks 2 months after LASIK.

• Confirm adequate (>65 mmHg) suction levels. [Use a Barraquer tonometer or pneumotonometer to check dilation of the pupil, dimming of the patient's vision, adherence of the suction ring, level of the suction pressure meter of the base unit, or pressure on palpation with fingertip (i.e., digital pressure).]

Management
• Abort the excimer laser correction (may further alter the irregular stromal bed and affect the final result).
• Leave the flap in place or replace it as precisely as possible into the stromal bed and leave it for at least 5 min.
• Monitor the eye weekly for epithelial ingrowth (more common after thin-flap complications).
• Consider a repeat LASIK procedure after 3 months using a deeper depth plate (180 or 200 μm).
• A free cap may still achieve an excellent outcome with laser treatment in the stromal bed and replacement of the cap.

CORNEAL NEOVASCULARIZATION Prolonged contact-lens use can cause neovascularization of the peripheral cornea. Vessels may be cut during the keratectomy step of LASIK and result in bleeding onto the stromal surface of the ablation bed

TABLE 11–2

Causes of Flap Complications after LASIK

Flap Complication	Mechanism
Perforated cornea	Absence or incomplete insertion of depth plate
Short flap	Obstruction of microkeratome path
Thin flap	Inadequate or lost suction
Irregular flap	Inadequate or lost suction
Button-hole flap	Inadequate or lost suction
	Ks > 48.0 D
	Mechanical theory of conservation of length leading to central corneal buckling and button-hole flap formation
Free flap	Ks < 41.0
	No microkeratome stop screw

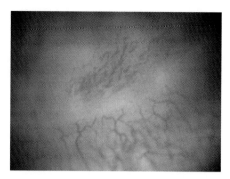

Figure 11–28 Interface blood immediately after LASIK.

(Fig. 11–28). Other etiological factors may be at work.
* large 9.5-mm keratectomy with Hansa-tome or other hyperopic rings
* a corneal scar or phlyctenule
* pterygium
* decentered keratectomy
* small cornea or microcornea

Prevention
* To avoid neovascularization, decenter the flap slightly inferiorly.
* Avoid using the large 9.5-mm ring of the Hansatome on small steep corneas.
* Anticipate bleeding in eyes with corneal scars that are associated with patent blood vessels.

Management
* Corneal neovascularization usually stops without treatment in a few minutes.
* Monitor any blood that extends onto the stromal bed to ensure that it does not move into the ablation zone of the laser.
* Absorb blood with a dry Murocel sponge as it progresses toward the ablation area.

* Temporarily arrest bleeding using direct pressure from the suction ring during the ablation process.
* Once ablation is complete, replacement of the corneal flap often tamponades further bleeding.
* Persistent corneal bleeds require additional treatment.
* To treat persistent corneal bleeding, locally apply a Murocel sponge soaked with Tobradex, 0.1% dexamethasone, 2.5% phenylephrine, or 0.5% aproclo-nidine.
* Apply filtered compressed air.
* Dry gently with a dry Murocel sponge.

PERFORATION OF THE CORNEA This extremely rare event may occur when LASIK is performed with the ACS (but without proper insertion of the depth plate) or any other microkeratome that allows insertion and removal of depth plates. The perforation becomes obvious when the microkeratome advances. Signs and symptoms of corneal perforation include:
* patient complaints of sudden pain
* the sudden appearance of intraocular fluid in the operative field
* a sudden drop in suction pressure of the suction ring
* the presence of extruded intraocular contents with a flat anterior chamber, peaking of the iris, or extrusion of the crystalline lens when reversing the microkeratome

Prevention
* This problem is best prevented by carefully inspecting the equipment before each case of LASIK.
* Use the "pre-flight checklist" advocated in training programs for technicians and surgeons to check the depth of keratome plate insertion before each use.

- Use the newer Hansatome with its fixed unremovable depth plate.

Management
- As soon as penetration is suspected, release the suction to minimize extrusion of the ocular contents.
- Gently remove the microkeratome from the eye.
- Place sutures across the corneal incision to stabilize the eye and then cover the cornea with a contact lens.
- Arrange for emergency referral to a surgeon who is comfortable with repair of the anterior segment.

POSTOPERATIVE PAIN Most patients do not experience pain following LASIK because of minimal epithelial disruption and the regularity of the post-LASIK corneal surface. Postoperative pain has many causes:
- epithelial defect
- dislodged flap
- toxic epithelial keratopathy
- residual pressure from suction ring/lid speculum
- infection (rarely)

Prevention
- Ensure that the procedure is as atraumatic as possible.
- Minimize the use of preoperative topical anesthesia to reduce postoperative epithelial toxicity.
- Administer 1 drop of a topical nonsteroidal medication to reduce the immediate foreign-body sensation.
- Advise patients to avoid rubbing or squeezing the eye because it may disturb flap position and cause significant pain.

Management
- Address any complaint of significant pain by performing an eye examination to ensure that the flap is in place and the epithelium is intact. (You will usually identify no major problems.)
- Administer a mild narcotic to assist with sleeping to reassure the patient.
- Provide topical nonsteroidal drops and lubrication drops to help control pain related to epithelial defects.
- Immediately treat the superficial punctate keratitis identified on the flap epithelium with generous lubrication.

EPITHELIAL DEFECTS Epithelial defects, which cause postoperative pain and a foreign-body sensation, are generally evident immediately after performing the keratectomy and most commonly form along the superior aspect of the keratectomy edge when using the Bausch and Lomb ACS (Rochester, NY) or the Hansatome (Fig. 11–29). The risk for epithelial ingrowth increases after stimulation of epithelial healing and growth begins. Etiology includes:
- anterior basement membrane dystrophy (ABMD) (Patients with ABMD commonly develop these defects; there is an even higher incidence for enhancements.) (Fig. 11–30)
- a history of recurrent corneal erosions (Patients with loose epithelium such as those with ABMD or a history of recurrent corneal erosions are best treated with PRK.)
- epithelial toxicity from topical anesthesia
- operative trauma/manipulation
- history of dry eye
- insufficient wetting of the corneal surface prior to passage of the microkeratome
- advanced age (Patients >45 years old tend to have a less adhesive epithelium to

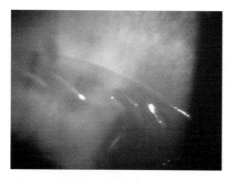

Figure 11–29 Loose epithelium with a defect along the flap edge immediately after LASIK.

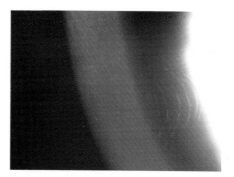

Figure 11–30 Typical appearance of the map lines of ABMD.

Bowman's membrane and frequently the epithelium is sloughed when the microkeratome is reversed.)

Signs and Symptoms
- significant pain
- prolonged visual recovery
- epithelial ingrowth
- flap melt
- infection
- LASIK interface inflammation (the "sands of Sahara")

Prevention
- Use topical anesthesia sparingly (once under the laser) to avoid any epithelial toxicity.
- Keep the corneal surface well lubricated to prevent epithelial irritation.
- Perform all surgical maneuvers with great delicacy to avoid any epithelial trauma.
- Use a modified technique if the patient has known ABMD.
- Do *not* mark the cornea.
- Perform a very wet (copious corneal irrigation prior to passage of the microkeratome) keratectomy to minimize friction between the depth plate and epithelium.
- To minimize sloughing of the epithelium, discontinue the vacuum at the completion of the forward pass of the microkeratome, and lift off the microkeratome and suction ring manually from the eye with the flap sliding out of the corneal shoot with minimal to no friction created over the epithelium.

Management
- Copiously lubricate the patient's eye and administer a topical prophylactic antibiotic drop to guard against infection daily until the defect heals.
- Small epithelial defects (<3 mm) generally heal quickly in 24 hr, so a postoperative nonsteroidal drop and a good sleep restore eye comfort.
- Treat larger epithelial defects with a contact lens, which reduces postoperative pain, lacrimation, and eyelid squeezing and generally remove it after 1 to 2 days.
- Alternatively, apply tincture of benzoine to the forehead and cheek skin and pull the lids together with paper tape to prevent blinking but do not apply gauze or a dressing beneath the tape. (This technique achieves minimal to no anterior-posterior pressure, only inferior-superior suspension.)
  ○ Follow patients with epithelial defects weekly for 1 month to monitor for epithelial ingrowth.

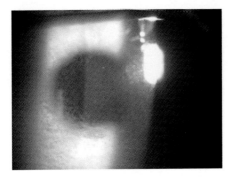

Figure 11–31 Grade 3 LIK with dense clumping of cellular material in the interface 3 days after LASIK. UCVA had dropped to 20/200 and BCVA was 20/50.

LASIK INTERFACE KERATITIS Laser interface keratitis (LIK), or the "Sands of Sahara" syndrome, presents as interface inflammation in the 24- to 72-hour postoperative period. The interface inflammation has a "sifted sand" appearance with a dusting of a powder-like material in the interface that generally is more dense centrally (Figs. 11–31 and 11–32). The rest of the eye usually unaffected with no conjunctival injection, anterior chamber inflammation, epithelial defects, or corneal infection (unilateral in 70% of cases). There are four grades of LIK (Table 11–3). Likely causes include:
• betadine
• benzene

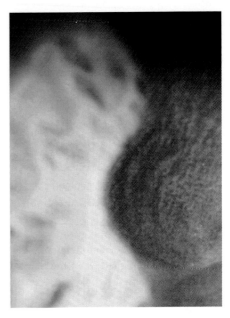

Figure 11–32 Grade 3 to 4 LIK. The circular inflammatory cellular material has formed along the rings of the broad-beam excimer ablation.

• BSS
• contaminants from eyelids
• contaminants on instruments (consecutive serial cases on the same day with same instruments and surgeon)
• corneal abrasions
• laser thermal effect
• lubricant
• meibomian gland secretions
• metallic debris
• talc
• topical medications
• bacterial endotoxin or exotoxin
  ○ endotoxins released from the cell walls of dead bacteria upon sterilization of improperly cleaned or stored instruments
  ○ exotoxins from patients with bacterial antigen loads from un- or undertreated blepharitis (isolated cases)

TABLE 11–3

Hatsis Classification of LIK

Grade	Interface	Topography	Vision
I	Partial	No change	Excellent
II	Complete	Irregular/shifts	Excellent
III	Complete	Irregular/shifts	Foggy
IV*	Complete	Irregular/shifts	Foggy

* And inflamed eye

Prevention

- Because causes of LIK remain unproven, prevention is difficult.
- Clean and autoclave instruments and, in particular, the keratome between cases.
- At the end of the operating day, clean, sterilize, and dry the instruments to remove all moisture (prevents an environment for bacterial colonization and active division).
- Analyze all loaner units or traveling microkeratomes for cleanliness.
- Remove potential endotoxins using a proper cleaning regimen (e.g., an absolute ethanol soak).
- Gently clean the packaged microkeratome blade before use to remove any surface debris that may stimulate inflammation.
- Immediately use topical steroid drops for the first few postoperative days to suppress any inflammation early.

Management

- Ensure sterility of cornea (no epithelial defects).
- Early identification of LIK allows the prompt initiation of topical steroid treatment, which may rapidly resolve the condition.
- More severe cases may take 4 to 8 weeks to resolve.
- Start topical steroids every hour and then slowly taper over several weeks.
- Treat severe cases with interface irrigation (reported as successful by some surgeons).
- Antibiotics have no obvious role.

INFECTION Infections or corneal ulcers are extremely uncommon after LASIK with an incidence of less than 1/5000 cases. Because the corneal epithelium protects against infection, the risk of infection is minimal once the epithelium is completely healed. The short time of exposure of the stroma and the lack of epithelial disruption minimize this risk. Infections begin as infiltrates in the area of an epithelial defect and, if left untreated, may progress into a typical corneal ulceration with infiltration, ocular inflammation, and pain.

Prevention

- Follow any patient with a postoperative epithelial defect daily to ensure that no infection occurs until the defect has healed.
- Use prophylactic antibiotics.
- Sterilize the microkeratome.
- Ensure good lid hygiene.
- Use antiseptic eyewash preoperatively.
- Wear talc-free gloves.

Management

- Assume that any corneal infiltrate associated with an epithelial defect after LASIK is infective and treat it immediately and aggressively.
- Perform corneal cultures (utility at this early stage of infection is controversial).
- Stop administering nonsteroidal medications and topical steroid drops.
- Instill topical fluoroquinolone every hour until improvement is noted.
- Lubricate the eye.
- Follow up with patient daily.
- If not resolved, switch to fortified topical antibiotics.

LASIK FLAP STRIAE Normally the striae are oriented horizontally with a nasal hinge and vertically with the superior hinge. Most flap striae occur within the first postoperative hour. Flap striae become more difficult to remove as the length of the postoperative course increases, and just 1 week postoperatively flap striae begin to become embedded in the corneal flap tissue (Figs. 11–33 and 11–34). Striae may be caused by

- misalignment of the corneal flap after flap replacement
- movement of the corneal flap during the first postoperative day

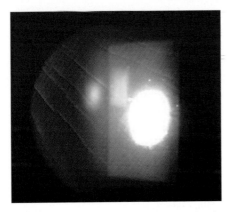

Figure 11–33 Retroillumination clearly demonstrates these severe striae caused by flap displacement 3 days after LASIK.

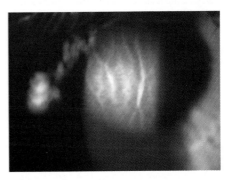

Figure 11–34 Severe striae associated with residual interface haze after LIK 3 weeks after LASIK.

- the "tenting effect" of the corneal flap over the ablated stromal bed

Prevention
- Reposition the flap with minimal manipulation once it has been replaced into the correct position.
- Instruct patients to avoid rubbing or squeezing the eye postoperatively.
- Instruct patients to wear eye protection 24 hours a day for the first week to prevent any eye trauma while the flaps heal.

Management
- Identify flap striae on the first postoperative day (imperative) because striae become more difficult to remove as the length of the postoperative course increases.
- Retroilluminate the fixation light and aiming beam through the dilated pupil to accurately localize the flap striae and identify microstriae in cases of unexplained reduction of BCVA.
- Treat flap striae that extend through the visual axis or induce regular or irregular astigmatism.

- Administer phenylephrine 2.5% (allows intraoperative retroillumination).
  ○ Mark the flap edge while viewing under the slit lamp.
  ○ Make no flap alignment markings.
  ○ Reflect back the flap.
  ○ Hydrate the stromal surface of the flap with BSS for 30 sec.
  ○ Replace the flap in the stromal bed and float it into position.
  ○ Leave the flap for 5 min to attach the stromal bed and dry the epithelial surface.
- Use the side of blunt forceps or a dry Murocel sponge to stretch the flap perpendicular to the striae.

DISLODGED FLAP Flap dislocation occurs in only 1/500 to 1/1000 of LASIK patients, usually because of some type of eye trauma or vigorous eyelid squeeze during the first 12 hr postoperatively. Vision becomes blurred and the eye becomes painful with an acute foreign-body sensation similar to the pain of a corneal abrasion. The incidence of epithelial ingrowth increases with both displacement and free caps.

Prevention

- Check the stability of the flap by ensuring that it is secure at the conclusion of the procedure by using the striae and blink tests (see p. 119).
- Wait 1 to 3 min after properly aligning the corneal flap and avoid excessive interface irrigation so that a strong seal may form.
- Advise patients to not rub or squeeze the eye.
- Provide eye protection for both day and night-time use.

Management

- Until flap replacement, lubricate the eye every 30 min with sterile preservative-free artificial tears to hydrate the flap and improve the discomfort.
- Patients usually keep the eye closed because of discomfort, or you may tape the eye shut until treated.
- Replace the corneal flap as soon as possible to avoid infection, reduce pain, and avoid permanent striae and damage to the flap (same procedure as for treating flap striae).

INTERFACE DEBRIS Interface debris often is present to some extent in most eyes following LASIK. Visual outcome is generally not affected and removal is unnecessary if the debris is inert. LASIK interface inflammation, however, does affect the visual outcome and should be differentiated from focal, noninflammatory interface debris. Following are examples of debris.

- lint
- red blood cells
- meibomian gland secretions
- metallic debris from blade
- dust
- rust particles from instruments

Prevention

- Interface irrigation during primary LASIK is the most effective method for reducing and potentially eliminating interface debris (removes ≥ 90% of the minute dust particles that are invisible under the laser microscope but visible postoperatively by slit lamp).
- Several other preventive measures help to avoid interface debris.
  - preoperative lid hygiene
  - washing the fornices
  - draping the lids
  - air filters in surgical suite
  - cleaning of all instruments between use to remove rust

Management

- If interface inflammation is suspected, follow the patient closely and begin administration of prophylactic topical steroids.
- Remove an interface contaminant that affects vision.
- Remove a large strand of lint that extends beyond the edge of the flap by pulling on it laterally with forceps.
- Remove debris that is completely under the flap using interface irrigation and flap repositioning (as in primary LASIK).

EPITHELIAL INGROWTH Reports indicate that 1.7% of eyes that undergo LASIK develop significant epithelial ingrowth that requires removal. However, refinements in the technique that delicately preserve the corneal epithelium have reduced this incidence to less than 1%. Epithelial ingrowth can occur in a number of patterns including lines, speckles, nest or pearls, strands, or sheets. Significant and persistent epithelial ingrowth often results in peripheral flap edge melt. Interface epithelial ingrowth may originate at three potential sites.

- stem cells peripheral to keratectomy edge (most common)
- isolated nest within the interface with no direct connection to the periphery (infrequent)
- passage through a defect in Bowman's membrane and flap stroma (rare; caused by trauma to these structures with direct communication of surface epithelium to the interface

Risk Factors
- preoperative risk factors
  - ABMD
  - a history of recurrent corneal erosions
  - advanced age
  - a history of ingrowth in the other eye
- postoperative risk factors
  - epithelial defects
  - flap edema
  - inflammation
  - repeat LASIK
  - flap slippage

Prevention
- Eliminate epithelial defects with LASIK (see Epithelial Defects section).

Management
- Identify the epithelial ingrowth by using one of several tests (Table 11–4).
- Consult Machat's practical grading system for epithelial ingrowth to guide the course of management (Table 11–5 and Figs. 11–35 to 11–37).
- Indications for treatment include the following.

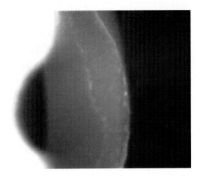

Figure 11–35 Grade 1 epithelial ingrowth.

  - greater than 2 mm of ingrowth from the flap edge
  - documented progression
  - associated flap melting
  - a disturbance of BCVA attributable to the ingrowth
- Mark the edge of the corneal flap using the slit lamp.
- Mark peripheral cornea alignment.
- Slowly dissect free the flap at its temporal margin.
- Gently fold the flap over its nasal hinge.
- Remove the epithelium from underneath the flap by peeling and scraping (use a dry Murocel sponge or blunt instrument).
- Remove the epithelium from the stromal side of the cap.
- Gently push back any epithelium hanging in the peripheral stromal bed.
- Replace the flap as for primary LASIK.
- Thoroughly irrigate underneath the cap to eliminate residual epithelial cells.

TABLE 11–4

Identification of Epithelial Ingrowth

Test	Finding
Tangential slit-lamp illumination	White to gray material under flap
Fluorescein staining	Pooling at the flap edge
Corneal topography	Surface irregularities
Retroillumination	Margins of sheets of ingrowth

TABLE 11–5

Machat's Epithelial Ingrowth Classification

Grade	Description	Treatment
1	Thin ingrowth, 1–2 cells thick, limited to ≤2 mm of flap edge, transparent, difficult to detect, well delineated white line along advancing edge, no associated flap changes, nonprogressive	No retreatment required
2	Thicker ingrowth, discreet cells evident within nest, ≥2 mm from flap edge, individual cells translucent, easily seen with slit lamp, no demarcation line along nest, corneal flap edge rolled or gray, no flap edge melting or erosion, usually progressive	Requires nonurgent treatment within 2–3 weeks
3	Pronounced ingrowth, several cells thick, >2 mm from flap edge, ingrowth areas opaque, obvious with slit lamp, white geographic areas of necrotic epithelial cells with no demarcation line, corneal flap margins rolled with thickened whitish-gray appearance, progression results in large areas of flap melting from collagenase release from the necrotic epithelium, confluent haze develops peripheral to the flap edge as flap pulls away leaving exposed stromal bed in contact with surface epithelium	Urgent treatment required with close follow-up Recurrences are more common because of the altered flap edges

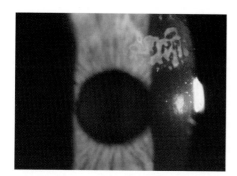

Figure 11–36 Grade 2 epithelial ingrowth.

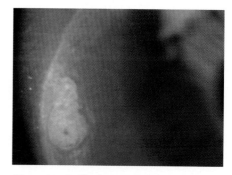

Figure 11–37 Grade 3 epithelial ingrowth.

ERRORS IN REFRACTIVE OUTCOME
Patients are disappointed if any significant refractive error remains after LASIK because they still depend on refractive correction (Table 11–6). Even a −12.00 D myopic will return for a −0.50 D enhancement, despite remarkable improvement in uncorrected vision. Although we are able to accurately program excimer laser ablation and perfect keratectomy techniques, the healing response of the cornea is the unknown variable with LASIK. Some patients may

TABLE 11–6

Errors in Refractive Result Following LASIK and Potential Treatments

Error	Comment	Enhancement
Hyperopia	Normal cornea	Hyperopic LASIK at 4 months
	Thin cornea	Laser thermokeratoplasty at 6 months
Myopia	1–3 D preoperatively	Myopic LASIK at 1 month
	3–6 D preoperatively	Myopic LASIK at 2 months
	6 D preoperatively	Myopic LASIK at 3–4 months
Regression	Wait for stability	Myopic LASIK
Astigmatism	Wait for stability	LASIK at 3–4 months

regress up to 3.0 D whereas others do not regress at all. Younger patients (<25 years) tend to regress and experience undercorrections whereas older patients (>45 years) regress less and experience overcorrections.

Prevention
- Ensure the accuracy and the stability of the preoperative refraction.
- Use a consistent LASIK technique with controlled stromal hydration and drying.
- Consult nomograms developed for LASIK that account for the degree of correction and age of the patient to minimize errors in the refractive predictability (Table 11–7).
  - Most myopia nomograms err toward undercorrection because myopia is generally less difficult to treat.
  - Overcorrect hyperopes by 10 to 20% because they tend to regress to emmetropia over 1 to 3 months.

- Carefully evaluate the technique that you choose, the geographic location of the laser center, the staff's attitude, and results to determine which nomogram is best for you.

Management
- A contact lens may manage any refraction as early as 1 week after LASIK, so that patients may return to full activities almost immediately.
- Topical steroids have little effect on refractive results.
- After achieving refractive stability, you may perform an enhancement procedure.
  - The greater the primary LASIK correction, the more postoperative time that is required to achieve full refractive stability.
  - Do not perform PRK over a LASIK flap because PRK may induce corneal haze.

TABLE 11–7

Probst LASIK Nomogram for VISX SmoothScan Laser

Amount of Myopia	Patient Age		
	<25 years	25–45 years	>45 years
<2.0 D	100%	100%	100%
>2.0 D	90%	86%	84%

CENTRAL ISLANDS Several situations lead to the formation of central islands.
- central accumulation of fluid
- inhomogeneous beam
- vortex plume with central shielding of successive pulses when using a broad-beam excimer laser

The presentation of central islands includes the following.
- loss of BCVA and UCVA
- irregular astigmatism
- monocular diplopia
- undercorrection

Although most central islands resolve by 1 month with no treatment or PRK.

Prevention
- Central island facto (CIF) software has been incorporated into the VISX laser to allow extra treatment to the central cornea to compensate for the central island effect of the broad beam laser.
- Scanning excimer lasers eliminate the risk of central islands.
  - Fluid does not accumulate centrally.
  - The vortex plume is not stationary.
  - Homogeneity of the beam with scanning lasers is not critical because of the smoothing or polishing effect of overlapping spots or slits.
- Remove any central accumulation of fluid by wiping the stromal bed during LASIK (alters overall stromal hydration and therefore affects the final refractive outcome).

Management
- Identify and monitor central islands with topography until they are stable in size and severity (Fig. 11–38).

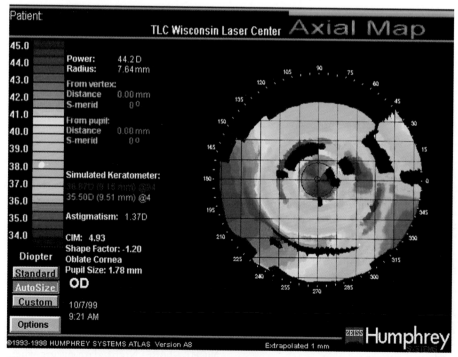

Figure 11–38 Corneal topography demonstrating a central island.

- Do not use refraction as an indicator of stability because it often varies considerably with each refraction.
- Treat a central island only if it causes subjective visual complaints or loss of BCVA.
- Topographic central island without patient complaints should not be treated just because the practitioner thinks it should be treated; treat the patient.
- Measure the size and height of the island with corneal topography (use the Munnerlyn formula to calculate the height of the island).

$$\text{height in microns} = \text{diameter}^2 \times \text{diopter height}/3$$

- Then correct the exact number of microns and diameter size of the island using the phototherapeutic keratectomy (PTK) mode on the VISX (Star or Smoothscan) or the Chiron 116 excimer laser.
- Alternatively, treat the refractive myopia in the PRK mode of the VISX laser but only for the first 50% of the ablation.
  ○ The Chiron 217 does not treat the central island well because the blending effect of the scanning laser does not allow the beam to be focused into the central area alone.
- Use a conservative approach because overtreatment results in a central divot, which creates irregular astigmatism and abrupt topographic changes over the pupillary axis (leads to multiple image formation or ghosting, which is difficult to correct surgically but may be treated with a rigid contact lens).

IRREGULAR ASTIGMATISM All patients have some degree of postoperative irregular astigmatism immediately, which gradually resolves a few weeks after the procedure. Persistent irregular astigmatism is now relatively uncommon but results in several undesired outcomes.
- reduced UCVA and BCVA

- visual distortion
- ghosting
- monocular diplopia

Prevention
- Proper surgical technique minimizes flap-related complications, such as striae.
- Check the homogeneity of the excimer laser beam regularly to ensure that the beam is smooth and symmetrical (irregular patterns are amplified during large corrections).
- Monitor hydration of the stromal bed (uneven wetting of the stromal bed can result in an irregular ablation pattern).

Management
- Postoperative topography, photokeratoscopy, manual keratometry, or even retinoscopy often uncovers some degree of irregularity that is related to some variation in corneal healing.
- Slit-lamp examination may reveal flap striae, LASIK interface inflammation, or corneal scarring which may result in irregular topographic patterns.
- Treatment of the flap striae and LIK (as described previously) dramatically improves both the symptoms and the topographic pattern.
- Corneal topography may demonstrate other irregularities of an otherwise normal cornea (e.g., central islands).
- Other irregular patterns are more difficult to treat because they require a customized ablation pattern.
- Topography-linked scanning excimer lasers offer the most promise for the treatment of irregular patterns.
- If all else fails, RGP contact lenses, if tolerated, are usually very helpful in reducing (if not eliminating) unwanted visual symptoms.

NIGHT GLARE Night glare occurs when the pupil dilates greater than the OZ of

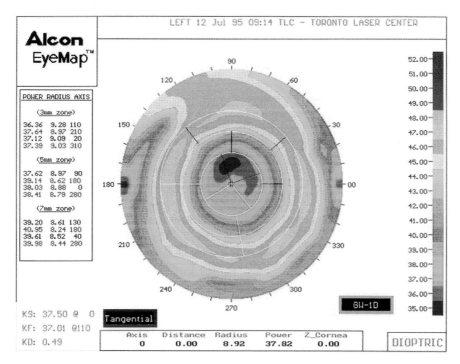

Alcon
EyeMap™

POWER	RADIUS	AXIS
(3mm zone)		
36.36	9.28	110
37.64	8.97	210
37.12	9.09	20
37.39	9.03	310
(5mm zone)		
37.62	8.97	90
39.14	8.62	180
38.03	8.88	0
38.41	8.79	280
(7mm zone)		
39.20	8.61	130
40.95	8.24	180
39.61	8.52	40
39.98	8.44	280

KS: 37.50 @ 0
KF: 37.01 @110
KD: 0.49

Tangential

Axis	Distance	Radius	Power	Z_Cornea
0	0.00	8.92	37.82	0.00

GW-1D

DIOPTRIC

Figure 11–39 Small OZ on topography 3 months after LASIK for a −10.0 D correction using a multizone algorithm on a broad beam laser.

the refractive correction (Fig. 11–39). Preoperative and postoperative night glare are more common in high myopes. Patients experience halos, starbursts, and reduced quality of vision. Although manageable in most patients, night glare may disable others.

Prevention
- Screen patient preoperatively for pupil size.
- Counsel patients with large pupils (>6 mm) in dim illumination about the potential risk of postoperative night glare.
- Treat patients with large pupils with larger-diameter ablation zones (≤9 mm); however, these lasers ablations remove significantly greater amounts of stroma so stromal thickness is the critical data point for determining candidacy.

Management
- Fortunately, most symptoms of night glare abate within the first year after the operation.
- Refinements in ablation profiles have resulted in significant reduction in the number of complaints of night glare.
  ○ Perform LASIK on the other eye.
  ○ Eliminate monovision.
  ○ Prescribe night-driving glasses (1.00 D).
  ○ Prescribe polarized lenses.
  ○ Use spectacle lens filters (shooter's yellow, lambda 540).
  ○ Instruct patient to use a night light in the car while night driving.
  ○ Initiate miotic therapy (pilocarpine 1/8%) to constrict pupil when night driving
- Surgical.
  ○ Retreat the eye by using a larger OZ and ablation zone.

○ Perform topography-assisted LASIK to same eye.

DECENTERED ABLATIONS Decentration of the ablation results in a residual refractive error (irregular astigmatism), which is associated with visual distortions and ghosting, particularly at night, and the patient may lose some BCVA. The patient's concerns are often more significant than expected for such a small refractive error. Decentered ablations have many causes.

• pharmacological pupillary dilation
• pharmacological constriction
• large angle kappa
• poor patient fixation
• wide flap hinge encroaching on ablation zone
• eccentric fixation

• treatment beam not coaxial with patient fixation beam (validate during instrument setup)

Prevention
• Always center excimer ablations on the pupil to minimize decentrations.
• Avoid pharmacological alteration several days before performing LASIK.
• To ensure centration on the pupil leave the suction ring on the eye but without active suction to control the position of the ablation completely.
  ○ Patients often have difficulty fixating on the fixation beam once the flap has been cut because the stroma does not provide a clear interface.

Management
• Detect decentration (obvious with postoperative topography; Fig. 11–40).

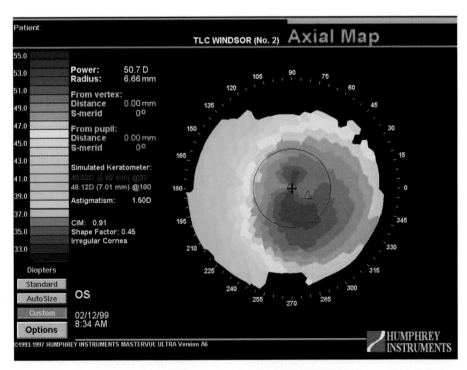

Figure 11–40 Decentered hyperopic ablation 4 months after hyperopic LASIK for a +5.0 D correction.

REFRACTIVE SURGERY: A COLOR SYNOPSIS

- Because the decentered ablation creates an irregular ablation pattern, treatment is difficult with a broad-beam laser.
- The refractive error is treatable and the flap is replaceable, these treatment options do not treat the edge glare effect from the sort edge of the ablation zone.
- A second ablation in the opposite direction of the original decentration has also been suggested but may result in a more irregular pattern.
- Topography-assisted LASIK (TA-LASIK) holds the most promise for decentered ablation because it treats the untreated area of the ablation zone.

LASER IN SITU KERATOMILEUSIS AS AN ENHANCEMENT PROCEDURE

Indications and Inclusion Criteria
- at least 1.00 D of myopia or hyperopia
- at least 1.00 D of astigmatism
- UCVA of 20/40 or worse

Risks
- overcorrection
- epithelial ingrowth
- flap striae
- infection
- pain

Preoperative Evaluation
- Ensure stable refraction.
- Ensure adequate corneal thickness using pachymetry.
- Perform regular topography.

Methods (Fig. 11–41)
- Mark flap edge at slit lamp.
- Place alignment marks on cornea.
- Lift flap before 6 months postoperatively.
- Recut flap at a deeper depth after 6 months.

- Peel back flap edge to minimize epithelial disruption.
- Perform excimer enhancement ablation.
- Refloat flap into position.
- Irrigate the stroma interface.
- To ensure centration on the pupil, leave that suction ring on the eye with the suction off to control the position of the ablation completely.
- Check alignment marks and gutter for alignment.
- Wait 1 to 5 min for adhesion to occur.
- Perform a blink and/or striae test.

Postoperative Management
- Monitor for ingrowth.
- Check refractive outcome.

Laser In Situ Keratomileusis after Radial Keratotomy
Indications and Inclusion Criteria
- myopia or hyperopia post radial keratotomy (RK)
- RK performed at least 1 year ago
- stable refraction
- regular astigmatism on topography

Risks
- unstable postoperative refraction
- decreased postoperative refractive predictability
- flap fragmentation
- epithelial ingrowth
- persistent starburst and night glare
- persistent diurnal variation
- potential increase in corneal anatomical instability

Preoperative Evaluation
- Ensure refractive stability.
- Measure early morning refraction.
- Make no more than eight radial incisions.
- The OZ should be at least 3.0 mm.
- Allow radial incisions to heal well.
- Verify no epithelial cysts.
- Ensure no reduction in BCVA from RK.

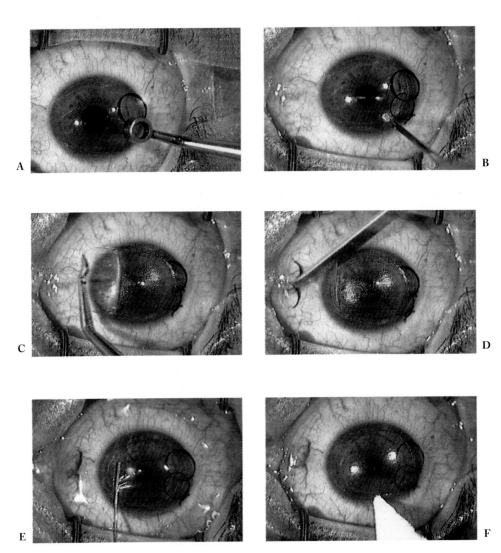

Figure 11–41 Technique of LASIK enhancement. (A) Flap edge is marked with alignment marks. (B) Flap edge is lifted. (C) Flap is grasped with nontoothed forceps and folded back. (D) Residual epithelial cells are scraped from the stromal surface of the flap and laser is then applied. (E) Flap replaced and the interface is irrigated. (F) Peripheral edge of the flap is dried and inspected to ensure good flap alignment.

Methods (Fig. 11–42)
- Use a 200-μm depth plate with ACS.
- Target slight myopia.
- Perform monocular treatment.
- Use extreme care with flap manipulation.
- Align flap and radial incisions carefully.

Postoperative Management
- Expect greater initial refractive fluctuations than with primary LASIK.
- Monitor patient for epithelial ingrowth.
- Do not lift the flap.
- Recut flap at 6 months for enhancements.

Laser In Situ Keratomileusis after Photorefractive Keratectomy
Indications and Inclusion Criteria
- myopia or hyperopia after PRK
- no corneal haze
- corneal thickness at least 450 μm

Risks
- persistence of superficial corneal haze
- epithelial defects
- epithelial ingrowth
- reduction in corneal anatomic integrity

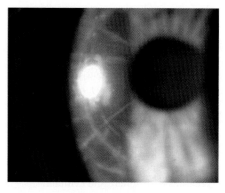

Figure 11–42 The peripheral edge of the LASIK flap can be seen going through the radial incisions of the previous RK.

Preoperative Evaluation
- Establish refractive stability.
- Ensure adequate corneal thickness.
- Ensure no corneal haze.
- Ensure no history of recurrent erosion after PRK.
- Confirm well-centered ablation with topography.
- Ensure no loss of BCVA from PRK.

Methods
- Use a 200-μm depth plate with ACS.
- Administer minimal topical anesthetic.
- Protect the epithelium with lubrication.

Postoperative Management
- Monitor patient for epithelial ingrowth.
- Refractive stability may take a few weeks to develop.

Laser In Situ Keratomileusis after Penetrating Keratoplasty
Indications and Inclusion Criteria
- residual myopia and astigmatism after penetrating keratoplasty (PK)
- sutures removed at least 1 year ago
- stable refraction
- regular astigmatism on topography
- adequate corneal thickness

Risks
- unstable postoperative refraction
- decreased predictability of postoperative refractive
- epithelial ingrowth
- dehiscence along graft edge
- induction of graft rejection
- greater incidence of enhancement

Preoperative Evaluation
- Measure stable refraction.
- Ensure regular astigmatism on topography.

Methods

- Wait 12 months after PK sutures are removed.
- Center suction ring on graft.
- Minimize suction time.
- Wait 2 weeks after PK before performing ablation.

Postoperative Management

- Prescribe topical steroids for 1 to 2 weeks to prevent rejection.
- Monitor for ingrowth.
- Wait 4 months before performing enhancement.
- Lift flap for enhancement.

Laser In Situ Keratomileusis after Automated Lamellar Keratoplasty

Indications and Inclusion Criteria

- residual myopia and astigmatism after ALK
- removal of sutures at least 1 year ago
- stable refraction
- regular astigmatism on topography
- adequate corneal thickness

Risks

- unstable postoperative refraction
- decreased predictability of postoperative refractive status
- epithelial ingrowth
- greater incidence of enhancement
- reduction in corneal anatomic integrity
- induction of irregular astigmatism
- loss of BCVA

Preoperative Evaluation

- Confirm refractive stability.
- Confirm no irregular astigmatism on topography.
- Ensure no loss of BCVA from ALK.

Methods

- Position the cut temporal to previous keratectomy.
- Use a 200-μm cut.

Postoperative Management

- Expect greater refractive fluctuations initially.
- Watch for ingrowth.
- Wait 4 months before performing enhancements.
- Lift flap for enhancement.

Laser In Situ Keratomileusis after Insertion of a Phakic Intraocular Lens

Indications and Inclusion Criteria

- residual refractive error after phakic IOL insertion
- posterior-chamber phakic IOL implantation
- refractive stability

Exclusion Criteria

- age less than 50 years
- extreme refractive errors
- thin corneas

Risks

- endothelial damage with anterior chamber IOL (ACIOL)
- dislocation of IOL
- crystalline lens or IOL in contact with posterior chamber IOL (PCIOL)

Preoperative Evaluation

- Ensure refractive stability.
- Perform regular topography.
- Wait at least 1 month after phakic IOL insertion before using a refractive laser.
- Keratectomy should be performed prior to ACIOL insertion, but refractive laser correction is still done 1 month later by lifting the flap.
- Rule out cataracts.

Methods (Fig. 11–43)

- Minimize suction time.
- Treat residual sphere and cylinder.

Postoperative Management

- Check IOL centration.
- Enhance as in primary LASIK.

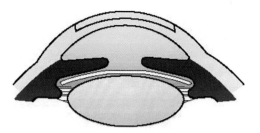

Figure 11–43 LASIK after insertion of a posterior chamber phakic IOL.

Laser In Situ Keratomileusis after Cataract Surgery

Indications and Inclusion Criteria
- refractive error after cataract surgery
- normal BCVA
- stable refraction

Risks
- dislocation of IOL
- additional loss of endothelial cells
- thin flap (because of poor suction)

Preoperative Evaluation
- Ensure refractive stability.
- Perform regular topography.
- Wait at least 1 to 3 months after cataract surgery.

Methods (Fig. 11–44)
- Ensure good suction.
- Use a 200-μm depth plate with ACS.
- Treat residual sphere and cylinder.

Postoperative Patient Management
- Check IOL centration.
- Enhance as in primary LASIK.

Topography-Assisted Laser In Situ Keratomileusis

Indications and Inclusion Criteria
- irregular astigmatism with primary LASIK
- decentered ablation zone after LASIK
- small OZ after LASIK

Risks
- reduced corneal thickness
- increased irregular astigmatism
- misalignment of centration or axis of custom ablation
- unpredictable results with central islands

Preoperative Evaluation
- Perform pachymetry.
- Estimate central K reading.
- Perform multiple high-quality topography.
- Send data to Technolas in Germany.

Methods
- Use a Hansatome flap to obtain the full effect of custom ablation.
- Ensure centration (critical).
- Ensure axis alignment (critical).

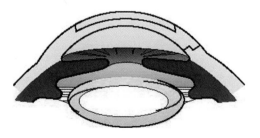

Figure 11–44 LASIK after cataract surgery or clear lens extraction.

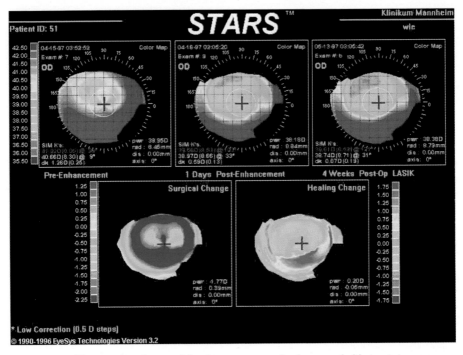

Figure 11–45 Topographic changes following treatment of a decentered ablation using topography assisted LASIK. (Courtesy of Micheal Knorz, M.D.).

Postoperative Management
- Expect longer visual rehabilitation compared with standard LASIK.
- Evaluate with topography (Fig. 11–45).

Suggested Readings

Doane JF, Koppes A, Slade SG. A comprehensive approach to LASIK. *Ophthalmic Nurs Technol.* 1996;15:144–147.

Machat JJ, Slade SG, Probst LE, eds. *The Art of Lasik.* Thorofare, NJ: Slack, Inc.; 1999.

Pallikaris IG, Siganos DS, eds. *LASIK.* Thorofare, NJ: Slack, Inc.; 1997.

Slade SG, Doane JF. LASIK: Laser in situ keratomileusis. In: Yanoff M, Duker JS, eds. *Ophthalmology.* London: Mosby; 1998:1–8.

Slade SG, Machat J, Doane, JF. Laser in situ keratomileusis: cornea. In: Kaufman HE, Barron BA, McDonald MB. *The Cornea.* 2nd ed. Newton, MA: Butterworth-Heinemann; 1998:1015–1036.

Wu H, Steinert R, Slade S, Thompson V, eds. *Refractive Surgery.* New York: Thieme; 1999.

CHAPTER 12

Custom Laser In Situ Keratomileusis with Wavefront Technology*

John F. Doane, Scot Morris, Andrea D. Border, Lon S. EuDaly, James A. Denning, and Louis E. Probst

CHAPTER CONTENTS

CURRENT OCULAR EVALUATION SYSTEMS AND LASER CORRECTION METHODS

Laser refractive procedures currently use only refractive data as the template for refractive programming of the laser. Although corneal topography systems contain descriptive data that could be incorporated into laser programs, early attempts to do so met with limited success. Results with topography-guided laser programs (e.g., Contoured Ablation Program; VISX, Inc. Santa Clara, CA) and topography-guided systems (TopoLink; Bausch & Lomb, Rochester, NY) have been limited. Wavefront technology attempts to overcome the limitations of these systems.

Limitations
• phoroptors and autorefractors
  ○ quantification of only sphere, cylinder, and axis of cylinder
  ○ lack of measurement of irregular astigmatism and other higher-order aberrations
  ○ limitation of resolution to 0.12 D
• corneal topography
  ○ extrapolation of height data from slope data by Placido disc or Humphrey topographer (Alcon, Fort Worth, TX) technology (leads to approximations of many of the mapped points)
• true height data obtainable but analysis limited to the cornea with slit-light systems (Orbscan; Orbtek but now Bausch & Lomb, Rochester, NY)

*The authors thank Greg Halstead, Thomas McKay, and Kevin Tausend of VISX, Inc., for their technical support and encouragement regarding this manuscript.

- accuracy of 0.25 D or 2 to 3 μm for corneal curvature and elevation data, respectively
- removal of only ~0.25 μm of tissue per pulse of an excimer laser

COMMON OCULAR ABERRATIONS

An *aberration* of a light ray is the deviation of light from the path that is predicted by standard first-order geometric optics. Seidel developed terminology that expresses the aberration of form as five sums, S_1 to S_5 (Table 12–1). For example, spherical aberration is eliminated when $S_1 = 0$. According to Seidel, no optical system may have all five sums equal to zero or have absolutely no optical aberrations.

Chromatic Aberrations
- A chromatic aberration is a deviation in the differential refraction of the color spectrum, but other aberrations that are unrelated to chromatic aberrations also occur.
- The cornea and crystalline lens each have a different refractive index for every wavelength of light.
- The eye focuses blue light (a short wavelength) in front of red light (a longer wavelength), which results in an imperfect point of focus.

- Chromatic aberration increases with the size of the pupil and increased distance between the light ray and the optical center of the cornea or crystalline lens.
  ○ The sharpest retinal image is produced when the pupil is 2 to 3 mm in diameter.
  ○ Pupils smaller than 2 to 3 mm degrade the sharpness of the retinal image by diffraction effects on the edge of the pupillary aperture.

Spherical Aberrations
- The converging power of a plus spherical lens increases as the lateral distance from the central ray increases.
- Rays at the edge of the lens are focused anterior to the focus of the central ray.
- No single, sharp point of focus exists for all light rays that pass through the pupil.
- The anterior surface of the cornea and the anterior and posterior surfaces of the crystalline lens cause spherical aberration in the human eye.
- The aberration is proportional to the square of the pupil size.
- The increase in spherical aberration and myopia (0.5–1.0 D) with pupillary dilation cause night myopia.

Oblique Aberrations
- These aberrations are identified after the correction of other types of aberrations (when off-axis light rays are less distinct than the light rays on the visual axis).

TABLE 12–1
Seidel's Sums of Optical Aberrations of Form

Classification	Aberration	Seidel's Sum
Spherical aberration	Spherical aberration	S_1
Oblique aberrations	Coma	S_2
	Radial astigmatism	S_3
	Curvature of field	S_4
	Distortion	S_5

- Oblique aberrations are difficult to define and measure.

COMA Coma is similar to spherical aberration but applies to off-axis light rays, which are distributed over a small area of the image rather than converging at a single point.
- The distribution of light rays resembles a comet.
- Coma is proportional to the square of the pupillary aperture and increases as the object moves away from the optical axis.

RADIAL ASTIGMATISM AND CURVATURE OF FIELD Radial astigmatism is also known as oblique astigmatism, marginal astigmatism, or astigmatism of oblique incidence.
- This property of all simple lenses is observed after removal of the spherical aberration and coma.
- A point off-axis is imaged as two lines at right angles to each other, each perpendicular to the chief (central) light ray.
- A multitude of points in a plane that are affected by radial astigmatism create curvature of field.
- Radial astigmatism and curvature of field negate each other when radial astigmatism equals curvature of field.

DISTORTION Inconsistent lateral magnification over the field of view leads to distortion.
- A pinhole camera is free of distortion because it has only central light rays.
- "Pincushion-" and "barrel-" shaped distortions (experienced when looking through a high-power lens) may result from distortion, depending on the configuration of the optical system.

Point-Spread-Function
- Diffraction occurs along the margin of the pupil.

- Limitations of the pupillary aperture cause light to spread, even in a perfectly focused system.
- The Fraunhofer diffraction image of a point object through a circular aperture has a bell-shaped distribution with oscillating fringes.
- The center portion of the pupillary diffraction pattern is a small circle called the Airy's disc.

Higher-Order Aberrations
- Wavefront technology identifies higher-order aberrations.
- These aberrations are then classified according to their Zernike order (up to the tenth order).
- Thibos and Hong (1999) have shown an increase in higher-order aberrations, specifically spherical aberrations, after myopic laser in situ keratomileusis (LASIK; Fig. 12–1).

Pupil Size and Optical Aberrations
- Image quality does not increase with pupils smaller than 2.5 mm because of diffraction effects from the pupil.
- Ocular aberrations increase as the pupil dilates, approximately offsetting the diffraction effects of a smaller pupil.
- With pupils larger than 5.0 mm, light spread increases because of greater aberrations present in the peripheral cornea and the increased amount of light that enters the eye from the peripheral area.

WAVEFRONT TECHNOLOGY

In the mid-1970s, Dr. Josef Bille, director of the Institute of Applied Physics at the University of Heidelberg, developed techniques to correct imperfect higher-order aberrations (or wavefront distortions)

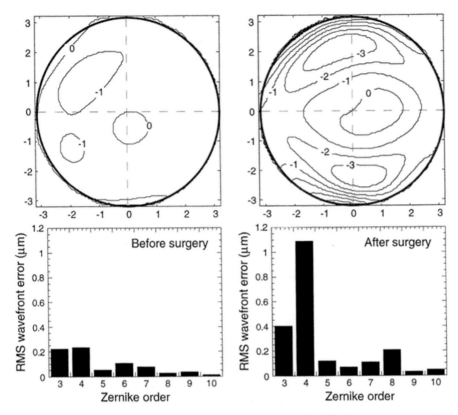

Figure 12–1 Normal eye the day before and the day after myopic LASIK. (*upper row*) Aberrations as related to the pupil. (*lower row*) The distribution of wavefront error by Zernike order. To emphasize the change in higher-order aberrations, residual spherocylindrical refractive errors were omitted from the analysis. The Zernike polynomial aberration of the first order is spherical error, the second order is regular astigmatism, the third order is coma, and the fourth order is spherical aberration. Other aberrations are measured up to the tenth order. Note the significant increase of third- and fourth-order aberrations along with the increase in fifth to tenth orders. (Courtesy of American Academy of Optometry. Thibos LN, Hong X. Clinical applications of the Shack-Hartmann Aberrometer. *Optom Vis Sci.* 1999;76:817–825.)

that entered telescopic lens systems from space. These techniques of wavefront technology used "adaptive optics," deformable mirrors were used to reform the distorted wavefront to allow clear visualization of celestial objects. According to Bille, 99.9% of the population undergoing refractive surgery have retinas that are capable of seeing 20/10, but the shape of their corneas does not permit such clear vision. Bille obtained the first German patents for wavefront technology in 1982 and 1986. In 1997, Bille cofounded 20/10 Perfect Vision, which designed and marketed a stand-alone desktop-sized testing device that includes an image acquisition device, monitor, computer processing unit, and keyboard.

The Shack-Hartmann Wavefront Analysis System

Wavefront analysis completely evaluates the entire optical system instead of limiting analysis to the confines of subjective or objective refraction and corneal topography. By measuring all optical aberrations of the ocular system, wavefront analysis potentially allows correction of these ocular aberrations.

Methods

- The system projects wavelengths of light as flat sheets or "wavefronts" into the eye, onto the macula, and through the entire optical system and then reflects the wavelengths back through the cornea.
- A charge couple device (CCD) video camera collects images within the acquisition module.
- In an optical system without aberration, the wavefront exits the eye as the same parallel flat sheets that entered the eye (Figs. 12–2A and 12–3A).
- In an optical system with aberrations, the flat sheets that entered the eye exit as irregular curved sheets (see Figs. 12–2B and 12–3B).
- The CCD video camera captures the returning wavefront and converts it to a color-coded acuity map (phase map or spatially resolved refractometer map) for points over the pupil area (Fig. 12–4).
  - The map is a translation of 100,000 data-point measurements taken every 20 μm over a 6-mm pupil.
  - The Shack-Hartmann data map demonstrates the raw light image that impinges on the CCD camera and demonstrates all the optical aberrations (Fig. 12–5).
- The technician obtains subjective patient feedback to determine potential uncorrected visual acuity (UCVA) by projecting an acuity chart similar to Snellen's onto the patient's fovea after application of the adaptive optics.

Limitations

- wavefront analysis
  - Tear-film abnormalities may significantly affect the quality of wavefront analysis.
  - Current Shack-Hartmann devices poorly define opacities because of the inability of the source testing light to reach the retina and reflect back to the CCD video camera.
  - Marked aberrations for corneal scars or keratoconus are very difficult to measure.
  - Miotic pupils are difficult to measure, may require pharmaceutical dilation, and provide data that do not represent the wavefront of the entire eye (Fig. 12–6).
  - Wavefront-sensing technology currently does not define the exact location of the pathology that is causing the aberration.
  - Techniques to create the "perfectly adapted optic" with spectacle correction or corneal or implant surgery to neutralize the pre-existing abnormal wavefront must be refined.
- retinal limitations for adaptive optics
  - Clinical or subclinical amblyopia may limit visual potential.
  - Some maculas may not have sufficient cone density to support 20/10 vision.
  - The directional sensitivity of the retinal cone receptors (Stiles-Crawford effect) limits the effect of light rays that do not enter the eye through the pupillary aperture.
- Retinal pathology or irregularities in high myopia or posterior staphylomas may limit the best vision possible.

Wavefront Systems for Refractive Surgery

THE 20/10 PERFECT VISION SYSTEM The first treatments using this Shack-Hartmann–style wavefront device were performed in the United States in early 2000. The system should be potentially commercially available in 2001.

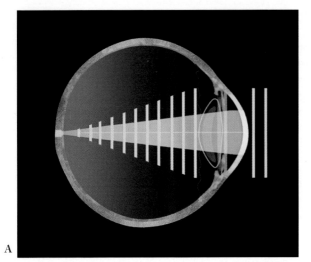

Figure 12–2 (A) Light reflecting from the retinal surface, traveling to the right, and exiting through the entrance pupil. This particular eye has no aberration, and the wavefronts are straight and parallel to each other.

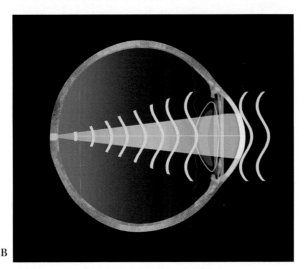

(B) Light emerging from an eye with significant aberration. The emerging wavefronts are curved.

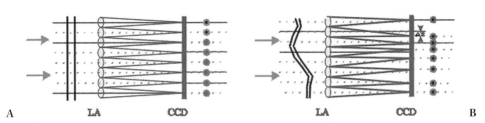

Figure 12–3 (A) Incident plane wave resulting in a square grid of spots. (B) A distorted wavefront causes lateral displacement of spots.

REFRACTIVE SURGERY: A COLOR SYNOPSIS

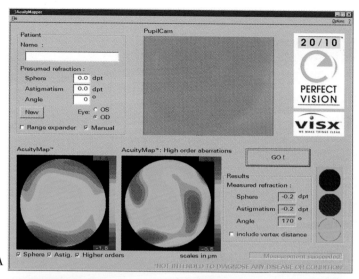

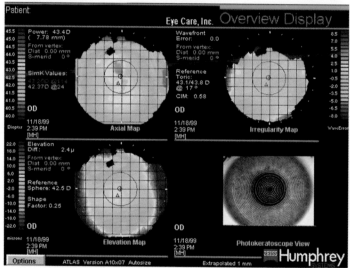

Figure 12–4 (A) A VISX 20/10 Perfect Vision Acuity Map of an unoperated "normal" eye. (*upper left*) Patient name, presumed refraction, and eye of regard. (*upper right*) A CCD picture of cornea and pupil. (*lower right*) The measured refraction via the wavefront reading for first order (sphere) and second order (regular astigmatism and axis). (*lower left*) The acuity map with sphere, astigmatism, and higher-order aberrations and the acuity map with sphere and regular astigmatism removed. The second map only describes the higher order aberrations. Note that the left map is scaled from −1.5 μm to +1.5 μm with most values from 0 (baseline reference plane) to +1.5 μm; the second map is scaled from −0.5 μm to +0.5 μm. In this example there are essentially no higher-order aberrations. These maps should be looked upon as contour maps. After taking the scale range in microns into account, widely spaced contours indicate an eye relatively free of optical aberrations whereas tightly spaced contours indicate a greater degree of aberration. (B) Humphrey corneal topography is provided for comparison.

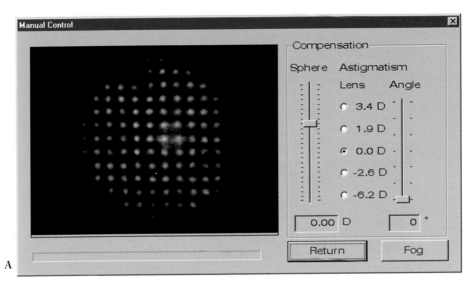

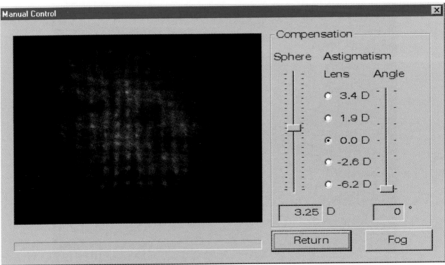

Figure 12–5 A Shack–Hartmann data map. (A) The central dots are relatively regular in size and alignment in the horizontal and vertical axis. (B) Dots are lost centrally and appear to be "moth-eaten." The overall irregularity of horizontal and vertical alignment of the spots of this eye indicate significant aberration.

- This system describes the refraction of the eye within 0.05 μm (five times more accurate than the excimer laser beam and approximately 25–50 times more accurate than phoropter-, autorefractor-, and topography-based systems)

- The device works with the VISX STAR laser as the VISX WaveScan Wavefront System.

CUSTOM CORNEA MEASUREMENT DEVICE
This Shack–Hartmann–style wavefront

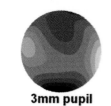

3mm pupil

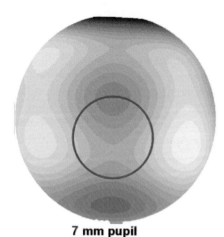

7 mm pupil

Figure 12–6 The observed map and data may also vary depending on the size of the pupil. The same examination at different pupil sizes demonstrates the contour changes within the defined 3- and 7-mm apertures.

directs the image to a low-light CCD linked to a computer. Dr. Theo Seiler and colleagues (University Eye Clinic, Dresden, Germany) developed the analyzer, and it is distributed by Technomed GmbH (Baesweiler, Germany) but will not be commercially available until 2001 or 2002.

- The Dresden analyzer evaluates the retinal image instead of outgoing light (unlike the Shack-Hartmann device).
- Use the analyzer with the Wavelight (Erlangen, Germany) Allegretto scanning-spot laser and scanning-spot laser from Schwind Eye-Tech-Solutions GmbH (Kleinostheim, Germany).
- Wavefront aberrations in the form of Zernike polynomials are computed from this data, which are integrated with preoperative corneal topography.
- An aberration-free ablation profile is calculated.
- The precision of the device allows for an objective measurement of spherical and cylindrical refractive error with an accuracy of better than ±0.25 D.
- The first three patients who were studied achieved uncorrected visual acuity between 20/12.5 and 20/10.

device may be commercially available in 2001 or 2002.

- This device is used with the LADARVision laser (Summit Technologies).
- All patients (5 of 5) achieved 20/16 to 20/32 vision in a 2000 U.S. Food and Drug Administration trial.

THE DRESDEN WAVEFRONT ANALYZER This analyzer is based on the Tschernig aberroscope, which was first described in 1894. A bundle of equidistant light rays are projected though the cornea, and an indirect ophthalmoscope measures deviation from the ideal pattern of all spots and

THE ABERROMETER/WAVEFRONT ANALYZER This Shack-Hartmann–type wavefront system was designed by Technolas GmbH (Munich, Germany).

- Use this analyzer in conjunction with the Orbscan topography device (Orbtek, now Bausch & Lomb, Salt Lake City, UT).
- Use with the Bausch & Lomb Surgical (Claremont, CA) 217 laser (the 217Z system for wavefront-guided LASIK, known as Zyoptix is currently available in Canada, Italy, and Germany)
- The Orbscan 3D corneal analyzer is linked to the ZyWave wavefront analyzer to provide maximum optical data.

• Most of the 200 eyes that have been treated at TLC The Laser Eye Center (Toronto) achieve better than 20/20 UCVA.

ELECTRO-OPTICAL RAY-TRACING ANALYZER

Tracy Technologies (Bellaire, TX) manufactures this analyzer, which uses the fundamental thin-beam principle of optical ray tracing to measure the refractive power of the eye on a point-by-point basis. No adaptive optics have been developed presently.

• This analyzer measures one point at a time at the entrance pupil rather than the entire entrance pupil at once (unlike the aberroscopes and Shack-Hartmann device) to avoid the possibility of data points crisscrossing with highly aberrated eyes.
• Semiconductor photodetectors detect the location where each light ray strikes the retina and calculates the difference from the ideal conjugate focus point, giving direct measurement of refractive error for that point in the entrance pupil.

SPATIALLY RESOLVED REFRACTOMETER

This analyzer is currently being designed, built, and tested by the Emory Vision Correction Center at Emory University (Atlanta, GA).

• Tests are completed in a relatively lengthy 3 to 4 min.
• Patients are directly involved in the testing (adds important subjective value).

EYE TRACKING

To achieve the maximum benefit from wavefront-derived custom LASIK, we must track the position of the eye so that the correct location is ablated. Any deviation from this exact position may lead to a significant decline in postoperative UCVA. Eye trackers that are currently available have several limitations that need to be addressed before the trackers are used successfully with custom LASIK.

Limitations

• The Bausch and Lomb 217 eye tracker has a relatively slow reaction time.
• The LaserSight LSX tracker may require the patient to maintain difficult head positions to get the tracker to work.
  ○ Intermittent tracker activation delays the procedure, potentially leading to stromal dehydration and overcorrection.
• The Autonomous Technologies tracker (now manufactured by Summit Technologies) requires pupillary dilation and predilation photographs that are time-consuming and cumbersome to obtain.

Suggested Readings

Dougherty PJ, Wellish KL, Maloney RK. Excimer laser ablation rate and corneal hydration. *Am J Ophthalmol.* 1994;118:169–176.

Liang J, Grimm B, Goelz S, Bille JF. Objective measurement of wave aberrations of the human eye with the use of a Hartmann-Shack wavefront sensor. *J Opt Soc Am A.* 1994;11:1949–1957.

Oshika T, Klyce SD, Applegate RA, Howland HC, El Danasoury MA. Comparison of corneal wavefront aberrations after photorefractive keratectomy and laser in situ keratomileusis. *Am J Ophthalmol.* 1999;127:1–7.

Thibos LN, Hong X. Clinical applications of the Shack-Hartmann Aberrometer. *Optom Vis Sci.* 1999;76:817–825.

Webb R, Penny CM, Thompson K. Measurement of ocular local wavefront distortion with a spatially resolved refractometer. *Appl Opt.* 1992;31:3678–3686.

CHAPTER 13

Clear Lens Replacement Refractive Surgery

John F. Doane, Scot Morris, Andrea D. Border,
and James A. Denning

CHAPTER CONTENTS

We evaluate refractive surgical procedures with five basic criteria.
- predictability [the percentage of eyes within a certain dioptic range from the target refraction (e.g., ±0.5 D)]
- accuracy [the percentage of eyes achieving a certain level of uncorrected visual acuity (e.g., 20/25 or better uncorrected)]
- stability of refraction over time
- safety [the percentage of eyes losing lines of best corrected visual acuity (BCVA) after a refractive procedure]
- quality of vision postoperatively

The clinician may find that this procedure is the best option; however, the clinician must evaluate the facts of each case and each patient's medical history to determine the most appropriate technique to use. The easiest and least invasive procedure may not necessarily be the best in terms of visual outcome.

Advantages
- high predictability and accuracy of refractive surgical result
- high level of safety
- very low incidence of lost lines of BCVA
- stability of postoperative refraction
- high quality of vision (does not alter the physiologic prolate corneal shape, thus avoiding potential iatrogenically induced aberrations)
- over 20 years of experience with technology (cataract surgery)
- a high level of experience and comfort with the technical aspects of the procedure for most surgeons
- greater predictability and postoperative visual quality for extreme refractive errors
- potential for treatment of eyes with low to moderate astigmatism (LASIK possible for any residual refractive errors)

Disadvantages
- loss of accommodation by the crystalline lens
- need for an intraocular surgical facility
- increased risk for intraocular complications
- endophthalmitis
- intraocular inflammation

- corneal endothelial damage
- retinal detachment
- blindness
- limitations of the low powers of intraocular lenses (IOLs) that are available for extreme myopia
- need for piggyback IOL insertion for extreme hyperopia

PREOPERATIVE CONSIDERATIONS

Indications
- early or frank crystalline lens cataract formation that may require cataract extraction in the near future
- certain presbyopic or prepresbyopic patients
- high hyperopia
- myopia
- thin cornea
- extremely flat myopic cornea (<40 D corneal power)
- extremely steep hyperopic cornea (>49 D corneal power)
- reasonable patient expectations

Patient Evaluation
- measurement of visual acuities (monocular and binocular corrected and uncorrected distance and near vision)
- refraction and retinoscopy
- quantification of BCVA
- determination of any visual loss because of cataract formation
- identification of opacity or irregularity of the crystalline lens (e.g., posterior lenticonus) from lens changes
- determination of the potential acuity measurement (PAM) (If the cornea is without pathology, a discrepancy between PAM acuity and manifest refraction BCVA suggests a crystalline lens cataract.)

- topography and keratometry
- comparison of corneal astigmatism with lenticular and globe astigmatism
- calculation of lens power
- determination of placement, number, and length of limbal relaxing incisions (see Chapter 8)
- slit lamp examination
- identification of corneal disease and anterior segment pathology (if present)
- evaluation of corneal thickness (must be consistent in area of limbal relaxing incisions)
- A-scan
  ○ preferably immersion instead of contact A-scan for greater accuracy
  ○ a noncontact laser A-scan (e.g., a Humphrey Eye Master; Alcon, Fort Worth, TX) may surpass an immersion A scan because it is extremely accurate to a hundredth of a millimeter
- lens power calculation (measurements of axial length and anterior chamber depth required, depending on the lens power equation)
- measurement of intraocular pressure (IOP) for baseline evaluation and comparison with any postoperative increase in pressure
- dilated fundus (rules out conditions that may affect surgical outcome)
- pseudoexfoliation syndrome (weak zonules)
- peripheral retinal pathology (e.g., tears, holes, or lattice)
- prophylactic laser photocoagulation to any retinal holes (reduces postoperative risk for retinal detachment)
- prophylactic peripheral barrier laser photocoagulation ("retinal cerclage"; 2–3 rows of 300–400 burns for 360 degrees in the peripheral retina) for high myopics
- focal treatment of any inner retinal pathology associated with increased risk for retinal detachment

- no detachments reported by Centurion up to 7 years postoperatively among 35 patients with axial lengths >26.5 mm
- preparation and patient completion of informed consent form

Lens Selection

SINGLE-PIECE POLYMETHYLMETHA-CRYLATE LENS The polymethylmethacrylate (PMMA) lens is the gold standard of IOL technology and has been used successfully for more than 20 years.

Advantages
- available in virtually all needed powers
- proven and dependable optics
- monovision a practical option
- excellent centration and stability within the capsular bag
- very inexpensive

Disadvantages
- need for limbal relaxing incisions for astigmatic treatment
- need for scleral tunnel approach
- high incidence of posterior capsular opacification (20–30%) requiring yttrium-aluminum-garnet (YAG) capsulotomy

FOLDABLE LENS Silicone, acrylic, and hydrogel lenses are currently available. Cataract surgeons prefer this lens because it allows small self-sealing (sutureless) incisions.

Advantages
- small size (≤ 3 mm) of corneal entry incision that is astigmatically neutral
- quickness of procedure
- ease of postoperative stabilization
- ability to reduce corneal or globe astigmatism by implanting a TORIC IOL (model no. AA4203-TL and AA4203-TF; Staar Surgical Company, Monrovia, CA)
- plate haptic design with cylindrical correction incorporated in its design

- currently available in 3.5 and 2.0 D powers that correct 2.4 and 1.4 D of corneal astigmatism (other powers under investigation)
- spherical powers available from 9.5 to 30 D
- lower incidence of posterior capsular opacification (2–3%; particularly for acrylic IOLs)

Disadvantages
- most experience with this lens gained over the last 5 years
- difficult management (if silicone oil required for complicated retinal detachment procedures) of movement with silicone lenses (after YAG laser capsulotomy)
- instability compared with the one-piece PMMA lens
- need for corneal refractive surgery to eliminate myopia (if patient unable to tolerate monovision)
- smaller range of IOL powers available for extreme high myopia and hyperopia compared with range for PMMA IOLs
- more expensive

MULTIFOCAL LENS The Medical Ophthalmics SIN40 lens (AMO ARRAY IOL; Allergan, Irvine, CA) is available in +10 to +30 D in increments of 0.5 D.

Advantages
- ability of both eyes to function at all distances (near, intermediate, and far)
- focused binocular visual function at each focal length
- less or no dependence on prescription spectacles postoperatively
- has all the advantages of other foldable IOLs

Disadvantages
- problems in mesopic and scotopic conditions

- glare or haloing
- inability to function in visually demanding situations
- patient dissatisfaction with subjective symptoms (e.g., night glare, distortions) that necessitates explantation and implantation of a monofocal lens

ACCOMMODATING INTRAOCULAR LENS C&C Vision (Aliso Viejo, CA) developed this lens, which is currently under investigation. This IOL focuses for distance when the patient fixates on distant objects and for near when the patient attempts to read by anterior displacement of the vitreous, which forces the lens optic more anterior thus creating a myopic refractive status for the eye and improving near visual function. The lens optic can move with vitreous pressure because of the optic's flexible arms.

LENS CALCULATION FORMULAS The length of the eye as measured by A-scan determines which formula you should use to calculate the parameters of the lens.
- short eyes
  ◦ Holladay II formula
  ◦ Hoffer-Q formula
- average eyes
  ◦ Holladay I formula
- long eyes
  ◦ SRK/T formula

SURGICAL CONSIDERATIONS

Contraindications
- all amblyopia or monocularities
- untreated peripheral retinal lattice degeneration or holes and tears or other inner retinal pathology (increases risk for retinal detachment)
- unreasonable patient expectations
  ◦ unwillingness to lose residual crystalline lens accommodation

◦ expectations of perfect near and distance vision

Patient Preparation
- Dilate pupil with 1% cyclopentalate and 2.5% phenylephrine 30 min before the procedure.
- Administer peribulbar block or topical anesthesia.
- Prepare skin and lid and draping in sterile fashion.

Standard Equipment
- keratome
- 0.12 forceps
- capsulorrhexis needle
- hydrodissection cannula
- viscoelastic substance
- lens manipulator or chopper
- phacoemulsification machine

Methods
- Create the clear corneal or scleral tunnel wound.
- Perform continuous curvilinear capsulorrhexis under viscoelastic substance control.
- Hydrodissect the lens material.
- Remove the lens using phacoaspiration, phaco cracking, or chopping (depending on the density of the lens material).
- Remove the cortex with irrigation or aspiration.
- Fill the anterior chamber and capsular bag with viscoelastic substance to protect the endothelium and intraocular structures.
- Insert and orient the implant into the capsular bag.
- Remove the viscoelastic substance with irrigation or aspiration.
- Pressurize the globe and check for wound leaks.
- Instill antibiotic and a steroid drop or ointment into the conjunctival fornix.

- Protect the eye with eyeglasses or a shield to prevent inadvertent trauma.

Alternative Treatments
- glasses or contact lenses (soft or rigid)
- excimer laser procedures [photorefractive keratectomy (PRK) or laser in situ keratomileusis (LASIK); see Chapters 9 and 11]
- laser thermal keratoplasty (for low hyperopes; see Chapter 10)
- phakic IOL insertion (high myopia and hyperopia; see Chapters 14 and 16)

POSTOPERATIVE CONSIDERATIONS

Results
- Expect at least 95% of eyes to be within ±0.5 D of targeted refraction.
- There is usually virtually no induced surgical astigmatism.
- Two to 4% of patient may want to have additional enhancement surgery for residual refractive error.

Postoperative Care
- topical antibiotic (4 times a day for 1 week)
- topical corticosteroid (tapered over 4 weeks)
- ocular shield for 1 week while sleeping
- follow-up visits (at 1 day, 1 week, 1 month, 4 months, and 1 year after surgery)
  - Check uncorrected distance vision.
  - Check near BCVA distance and near vision with manifest refraction.
  - Check IOP.
  - Check lens position.
  - Assess anterior segment cell and flare.
  - Assess vitreous humor and posterior pole.

Complications and Management
- poor refractive outcome (enhancement possible)
- lack of tolerance for monovision or multifocal vision (prepare for enhancement)
- retinal detachment
  - 1 to 6% annual rate after extracapsular cataract extraction
  - 0.7% annual rate with no surgical intervention for high myopes (>10 D)
  - High hyperopes have a much lower rate because of the different peripheral vitreoretinal interactions in short eyes.
- endophthalmitis
  - This complication occurs in less than 0.1% of cataract surgery patients.
  - Promptly tap anterior chamber or vitreous humor for culture.
  - Promptly administer intravitreal broad-spectrum antibiotic coverage for gram negative and gram positive organisms.
  - Adjust the antimicrobial regimen as soon as speciation and sensitivities are complete.
- expulsive choroidal hemorrhage
  - Ensure that the wound is water tight to prevent extrusion of intraocular contents.
  - Attempt scleral cut downs for choroidal drainage.
- retrobulbar hemorrhage with retrobulbar anesthesia
  - If extensive, postpone the procedure to allow clearance of hemorrhage.
  - Be alert to increased risk for complications from inappropriately high posterior vitreous pressure particularly in high hyperopes with small eyes.
- torn posterior capsule
  - If vitreous presents, select and place the acrylic or PMMA IOL in the sulcus after reducing the IOL power 0.5–1.0 D if safe to do so.
- posterior capsule opacification

- If BCVA decreases or subjective symptoms are present, manage with YAG laser capsulotomy.
- endothelial damage or decompensation
  - Use viscoelastic substances and a gentle surgical technique to protect the endothelium.
  - If mild damage occurs, instill 5% hypertonic drops or ointment.
  - Administer topical corticosteroid drops early in the postoperative period to help minimize insult.
  - If chronic damage or decompensation leads to bullous keratopathy, penetrating keratoplasty may be necessary to restore the corneal clarity.
- wound dehiscence
  - Ensure proper wound construction.
  - Confirm a tight water seal at the end of the procedure.
- residual refractive error
  - Properly understand lens formulas and how to use them.
  - Have experience in dealing with a particular lens and in treating short and long eyes.
  - Manage with contacts or spectacles, corneal refractive surgery, or IOL implant exchange.

Enhancements and Secondary Procedures
- corneal refractive surgery (for residual refractive error)
- incisional keratotomy
- radial keratotomy
- astigmatic keratotomy
- limbal relaxing incisions [often in conjunction with clear lens replacement (CLR) or cataract surgery]
- laser refractive procedures
- PRK
- LASIK [preferred method after refractive lensectomy (RL) or phakic IOL insertion]
- laser thermokeratoplasty
- an intracorneal ring (Intacs; KeraVision, Fremont, CA)

Clear Lens Extraction Plus Laser In Situ Keratomilieusis

This combined technique, also known as bioptics, was introduced by Dr. Roberto Zaldivar of Argentina for use with phakic IOLs (Figs. 13–1 and 13–2).

Advantages
- fully corrects spherical error with CLR
- fully corrects any residual spherical error or astigmatism with LASIK
- preserves high visual quality
- keeps risk for loss of BCVA minimal for even extreme corrections

Disadvantages
- need for two procedures at least 1 month apart
- risk for complications with both procedures
- potential IOL movement when suction applied during LASIK keratectomy
- expensive technology required

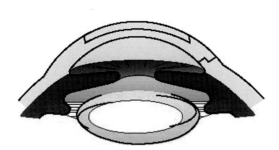

Figure 13–1 The bioptic concept as applied to CLR with LASIK. The benefits of both procedures can be combined to correct virtually any refractive error.

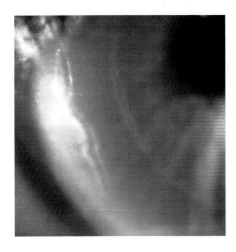

Figure 13–2 The two incisions are visible in the right eye. The more linear, vertical 3.2-mm incision on the left is from the refractive lensectomy (RL). The more central, round incision on the right is from the LASIK keratectomy edge.

Suggested Readings

Allen HF, Bangiaracine AB. Bacterial endophthalmitis after cataract extraction. *Arch Ophthalmol.* 1974;91:3–7.

Christy NE, Lall P. A randomized controlled comparison of anterior and posterior periocular injection of antibiotic in the prevention of postoperative endophthalmitis. *Ophthalmic Surg.* 1986;17:715–718.

Doane JF, Nordan LT, Baker RN, Slade SG. Basic tenets of lamellar refractive surgery. *Ocul Surg News.* 1996;Jul 1:31.

Goldberg MF. Clear lens extraction for axial myopia: an appraisal. *Ophthalmology.* 1987;94: 571–582.

Lindstrom RL. Retinal detachment in axial myopia. *Dev Ophthalmol.* 1987;14:37–41.

Miller KM, Glasgow BJ. Bacterial endophthalmitis after sutureless cataract extraction. *Arch Ophthalmol.* 1993;111:377–379.

Praeger DL. Five years' follow-up in the surgical management of cataracts in high myopia treated with the Kelman phacoemulsification technique. *Ophthalmology.* 1979;86: 2024–2033.

Werblin TP. Clear lens/cataract extraction for refractive purposes. In: Elander R, Rich LF, Robin JB, eds. *Principles and Practice of Refractive Surgery.* Philadelphia: WB Saunders; 1997: 449–458.

CHAPTER 14

The NuVita Angle Supported Phakic Intraocular Lens

Andrea D. Border, John F. Doane, Scot Morris, and James A. Denning

CHAPTER CONTENTS

The original Baikoff anterior chamber intraocular lens (AC IOL) design that was first introduced in 1989 included an anterior vault, 4.5-mm optic diameter, and four-point haptic fixation. This phakic IOL was essentially a modification of the successful Kelman AC IOL used for aphakic eyes. The next generation of the Baikoff IOL (NuVita MA20; Bausch & Lomb, Rochester, NY), which is now being used, has an improved footplate design to decrease pupil ovalization and an increased optic zone from 4.0-mm to 4.5-mm (5.0-mm optic width overall). Peripheral detail treatment (PDT) has been used to modify the 5.0-mm optic edge to decrease edge glare and halos.

Advantages
- decreased potential aberrations (corneal contour left prolate)
- accommodation left intact
- almost complete reversibility
- lower cost than excimer laser procedures

- greater success than corneal refractive procedures for correcting higher refractive errors

Disadvantages
- potential intraocular complications
  - endophthalmitis
  - corneal endothelial damage
  - intraocular inflammation
  - cataract
- fewer study results
- need for an intraocular surgical facility
- current inability to correct astigmatism

PREOPERATIVE CONSIDERATIONS

Indications
- extreme myopia or hyperopia (myopia > −10 to −12 D; hyeropia > +4 to 6 D)
- cases in which laser in situ keratomileusis (LASIK) is contraindicated

Inclusion Criteria
- AC depth greater than 3.0 mm
- patient age 25 to 45 years old
- patient comfort with surgical risks
- reasonable patient expectations about results

Patient Evaluation
- Determine monocular and binocular, corrected and uncorrected, distance and near visual acuity.
- Measure manifest and cycloplegic refraction.
  - Do not rely on patient's habitual spectacle power as the manifest refraction because high myopes are frequently over minused (see Chapter 4).
- Perform topography and keratometry.
  - Ensures that astigmatic power and axis coincide with manifest refraction astigmatic power and axis.
  - Helps to plan placement of limbal relaxing incisions (LRIs) to correct astigmatism when implanting the phakic IOL (see Chapter 8).
- Perform a slit-lamp examination (rules out or identifies corneal disease and anterior segment pathology or inflammation).
- Measure the horizontal white-to-white limbal distance (add 0.5–1.0 mm to corneal diameter to determine the overall size of the NuVita IOL).
- Measure the length of the eye with an A-scan.
  - This measurement is not necessary for phakic IOL implantation (phakic IOL is an *additional* lens, not a replacement but may be helpful later for future cataract extraction and determination of AC depth).
  - Use a current applanation or immersion A-scan [identifies AC depth (>3.0 mm is needed) to determine the safety of phakic IOL implantation].
- Measure intraocular pressure (IOP) (21 mmHg is a risk factor for glaucoma).
- Perform gonioscopy (rules out AC angle abnormalities such as peripheral anterior synechiae, which could complicate implantation of the phakic IOL into the angle).
- Examine the dilated fundus.
  - Rules out any severe, progressive, or inflammatory vitreal or retinal pathology.
  - Identifies any peripheral retinal degeneration, holes, or tears (may be safely treated with focal or barrier laser photocoagulation before phakic IOL implantation).
- Perform ultrasound biomicroscopy (UBM) (obtains more accurate measures of AC depth and exact configurations of AC anatomy).
- Have several different-sized implants on hand so they may be exchanged quickly if necessary.
- Determine the amount of diopter power needed.
  - Gather data obtained during patient evaluation.
  - Consult the nomogram or formula provided by the manufacturer of the AC phakic IOL that is to be implanted [e.g., the NuVita phakic IOL (model MA20) nomogram by Bausch & Lomb] (Fig. 14–1).

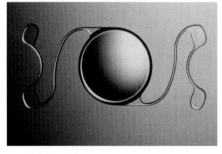

Figure 14–1 The NuVita phakic intraocular lens (model MA20), an AC, angle-fixated phakic IOL.

SURGICAL CONSIDERATIONS

Relative Contraindications
- amblyopia
- monocularity
- iris atrophy
- untreated peripheral retinal lattice degeneration, holes, or tears
- endothelial cell count less than 2500 cells/mm^2 (procedure itself may cause a loss of 8–10%, followed by 1% per year)
- glaucoma

Absolute Contradictions
- inflammation of anterior or posterior segment
- corneal dystrophy or scars that reduce best corrected visual acuity
- iris rubeosis
- significant or progressive retinal pathology
- microphthalmia
- cataracts
- regular patient participation in violent or high-contact sports (e.g., boxing, karate, and football)

Equipment
- forceps
- steel or diamond keratome
- viscoelastic substance (ensures adequate formation of the AC by protecting the endothelium)
- goniolenses (ideally, Thorpe- and Zeiss-type goniolenses)
- Kuglen hook (recommended but optional)
- cystitome (recommended but optional)

Methods
- Gently massage the eye or place a Honan balloon on the eye for a 5 to 10 min to soften it.
- Measure (or remeasure) the white-to-white corneal limbal distance.
- Instill several drops of pilocarpine 1 to 4%.
- Topical (proparicaine 0.5%) or local anesthesia (lidocaine 2%) is preferred, but general anesthesia may be used.
- Create a temporal, self-sealing, 5.5-mm clear corneal incision that has a groove and a 1.5-mm tunnel into the AC.
- Immediately insert a viscoelastic substance (Healon or Provisc; Alcon, Fort Worth, TX or Occucoat; STAAR Surgical Co., Monrovia, CA), but avoid introduction of any viscoelastic substance behind the iris.
- Position yourself to the side of the patient's head.
- Hold the closest (superior) edge of the implant with forceps.
- Snake the leading (lower or *farthest*) haptic into the AC (do *not* touch the anterior lens capsule or the corneal endothelium).
- Continue to hold the superior (closest) edge of the implant with forceps.
- Guide the implant across the iris until both ends of the lower (leading) haptic are in the angle.
- Ensure that the pupil is still round and not deformed or ovalized.
- Verify that the trailing (closest) haptic is still outside the AC (if already inside the eye, the implant is too small).
- Grasp the elbow of the trailing haptic with forceps to push the lens across the AC without tucking the iris (may avoid full insertion of the implant into the eye if the IOL is too small) (Fig. 14–2).
- Place a Thorpe-type goniolens and a viscous-substance cushion on the cornea.
- Carefully ensure there is no iris tuck (causes ovalization of the pupil) (Fig. 14–3).
- Resolve any iris tuck before placing the remaining (trailing) haptic in the angle (reduces the risk for hyphema).
- Grasp the trailing haptic just under the edge of the right footplate using forceps.
- Gently press the right haptic into the eye (direct it downward so that it springs back under the cornea).

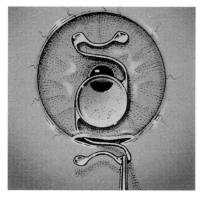

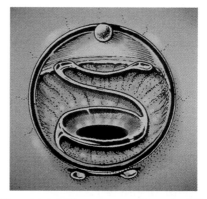

Figure 14–2 The surgeon may prefer to grasp the elbow of the trailing haptic with forceps to push the lens across the AC, taking care not to tuck the iris with the IOL.

Figure 14–3 A Thorpe-type goniolens should be placed on the eye with a viscous-substance cushion to make sure no iris tuck is present after the leading haptic has been positioned in the angle.

- Retract the posterior edge of the incision with a Kuglen hook.
- Insert the left end of the trailing haptic with forceps and allow the haptic to spring back under the posterior lip of the wound.
- Place a fork-shaped or collar-button IOL manipulator into the curve of the bridge between the two footplates of the trailing haptic.
- Alternatively, a surgeon may push *both* footplates into the AC and under the posterior lip of the wound (avoids the need for another hand to pull the wound open and avoids placing forceps into the eye a second time).
- Again, ensure there is no iris tuck by using a Zeiss-type goniolens to visualize the trailing haptic ends.
- Verify that the leading haptics have not been displaced by insertion of the trailing haptics using a Thorpe-type goniolens and viscous substance cushion.
  ○ If the leading haptics are positioned incorrectly, use a lens hook (or cystitome) to retract and reposition them.
  ○ If the trailing haptics are positioned incorrectly, use a Kuglen hook to push

the haptic away from the angle and then release it (Fig. 14–4).
- Again, verify correct positioning of the haptics using a goniolens.
- Place an optional iridotomy one fourth of the distance from the angle to the center

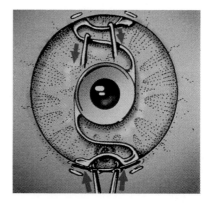

Figure 14–4 If the trailing haptics are positioned incorrectly or iris tuck is present (as seen by the Zeiss-type goniolens), use a Kuglen hook to push the haptic away from the angle and then release. If the leading haptics are misplaced or there is iris tuck, use a cystitome to retract and reposition the leading haptic.

of the pupil and midway between the ends of the trailing (closest) haptics.

- Place one or two sutures across the wound (do not tie them).
- Gently and slowly irrigate and aspirate viscoelastic substance to avoid displacing the implant.
- Tie the sutures.
- Make a final gonioscopic evaluation after closing the incision.

Potential Alternative Treatments

- glasses
- contact lenses (soft or rigid-gas permeable)
- LASIK (see Chapter 11)
- photorefractive keratectomy (PRK; see Chapter 9)
- clear lens replacement (see Chapter 13)

POSTOPERATIVE CONSIDERATIONS

Mild Complications

- inflammatory reactions
- anterior subcapsular vacuoles
- early pupillary block
- cataracts

Moderate Complications

- halos and glare (subjectively mild, moderate, or severe)
- ovalization or distortion of the pupil
  ○ progressive or nonprogressive
  ○ 7 to 30% overall incidence
  ○ caused by an IOL that is too large
- endothelial cell count reduction (usually parallels normal cell count reduction of 0.5–1.0% per year but may be progressive)
- footplate caught in peripheral iridectomy
- implant displacement or rotation (usually apparent within 3–18 months)
- potential glaucoma from long-term angle damage

Severe Complications

- endophthalmitis
- retinal detachment (no evidence of increased risk with phakic IOL insertion)

Prevention and Management of Complications

- Most inflammatory reactions, early pupillary block, and anterior subcapsular vacuoles resolve spontaneously with little or no intervention.
- Hypotony and early pupillary block associated with Seidel's sign that do not resolve in 24 hr require reopening the corneal incision and resuturing the wound.
- glare or halos
  ○ Most complaints decrease by an estimated 33% over the first 1 to 3 months, or the patient begins to tolerate the symptoms.
  ○ Prescribe low-dose pilocarpine (0.125–1%) at night.
  ○ Explant the lens if symptoms are persistent or severe.
- ovalization or distortion of the pupil
  ○ Carefully monitor the iris during implantation.
  ○ Carefully choose the size of the implant.
  ○ Do not push too hard on the iridocorneal angle with the footplates.
  ○ Move the lens farther forward if distortion is too progressive.
- endothelial cell count reduction
  ○ Maintain formed AC with viscoelastic substance to avoid touching endothelium.
  ○ Select the proper size of implant (an IOL that is too small may lead to pseudophakodonesis, which causes significant direct contact and mechanical trauma to endothelium).
  ○ Explant lens if lens reduction is too progressive.
- footplate caught in the peripheral iridectomy
  ○ Do *not* place the iridectomy below the area covered by the upper lid.

- ◦ Surgically correct by repositioning the haptic.
- Implant displacement or rotation requires surgical repositioning.
- Use prophylactic antibiotics intraoperatively to prevent endophthalmitis.
- retinal detachments
  - ◦ Pretreat suspicious areas of lattice degeneration with focal laser or barrier laser around the full periphery.
  - ◦ Treat with photocoagulation or cryopexy.

Enhancements and Secondary Procedures

LASER IN SITU KERATOMILEUSIS Perform LASIK to correct residual spherical or cylindrical error (see Chapter 11 for procedural details). With the NuVita AC IOL, perform the keratectomy of the LASIK before inserting the phakic IOL because the proximity of the AC lens to the endothelium may result in endothelial damage when the cornea is flattened during the keratectomy. Jose Guell named this approach the "adjustable refractive surgery" or ARS concept. After inserting the NuVita lens and refraction is stable, the surgeon lifts the flap and performs the refractive excimer laser "enhancement."

LIMBAL RELAXING INCISIONS Create LRIs to correct residual astigmatism of 2.50 to 3.00 D. Place LRIs simultaneously with implantation of a phakic IOL. (See Chapter 8 for details about the procedure.)

PHAKIC IOL EXCHANGE AND POSSIBLE SIMULTANEOUS REMOVAL OF THE NATURAL LENS If the NuVita phakic IOL causes disabling visual problems (e.g., glare or halos) or persistent ocular complications (e.g., progressive endothelial cell loss or cataracts), then the surgeon should remove it. In many cases, repositioning or replacement of the lens with a better-sized one

corrects the problem. With a cataract, the NuVita IOL needs to be removed and a standard cataract extraction procedure performed followed by insertion of an IOL in the capsular bag.

Methods

- The most common choice is a local ocular anesthetic (lidocaine 2–4%), but general anesthesia may also be used.
- If only phakic IOL explantation is required (no cataract), then instill two drops of pilocarpine.
- Inject viscoelastic into the eye and continue as noted below.
- If planning explantation of the phakic IOL and simultaneous removal of the natural lens, do the following.
  - ◦ Induce preoperative mydriasis.
  - ◦ Remove the cataract through a 3-mm clear corneal incision to maintain the stability of the AC.
  - ◦ Proceed with the capsulorrhexis using forceps.
  - ◦ Evulse the nucleus.
  - ◦ Clean and aspirate the cortex (should be easy because the natural lens has a soft texture).
  - ◦ Wait until the *end* of the procedure to extend the incision for explanting the IOL or implanting a new, lower power, posterior chamber implant.
- Depending on the quality of the capsulorrhexis, fix the implant in the capsular sac or to the ciliary sulcus.
- Perform paracentesis of the AC at the initial point of incision.
- Inject sufficient viscoelastic substance into the AC in front of the implant to deepen the AC.
- Simultaneously depress the lower lip of the paracentesis to allow aqueous outflow.
- Extend the corneal incision to 6 mm with a scalpel or diamond knife (if planning to perform simultaneous clear lens replacement surgery with phakic IOL extraction,

wait until the *end* of the procedure to extend the corneal incision).

- Dislodge the implant from the iridocorneal angle opposite the incision with forceps.
- Replace or remove the implant, and completely remove all viscoelastic substance.
- Close the corneal incision (without leaks) with 10-0 nylon sutures.

Postoperative Care

- Prescribe combination antibiotic/steroid drops (Tobradex; Alcon) four times a day on a slow taper that decreases by one drop a day per week.
- Instruct the patient to wear an ocular shield at night for 5 to 7 days.
- Prescribe preservative-free artificial tears for 1 to 2 weeks, as needed.

Follow-Up

- Examine patients at day 1; weeks 1, 3, and 6; and 12 months.
- Monitor endothelial cell count and compare with preoperative measurement at 3, 6, and 12 months.
  - The minimum threshold for explantation of a phakic IOL is a 50% decrease in endothelial cell count because chances are good for maintaining corneal trans-

parency throughout life with 50% of original endothelial cell count.

- Monitor IOP, all anterior segment parameters, the presence or absence of inflammation, the condition of the pupil, the iris, the iridocorneal angle, and the clarity of the natural lens.
- Monitor refraction (if refractive error significantly affects visual performance, consider phakic IOL exchange).
- Monitor the posterior pole and peripheral retina annually.

Suggested Readings

Baikoff GD. Refractive phakic intraocular lenses. In: Elander R, Rich LR, Robin JB, eds. *Principles and Practice of Refractive Surgery.* Philadelphia: WB Saunders Company; 1997: 435–447.

Baikoff G, Arne JL, Bokobza Y, et al. Angle fixated anterior chamber phakic intraocular lens for myopia −7 to −9. *J Refract Surg.* 1998;14: 282–293.

Wu HK, Thompson VM, Steinert R, Hersh PS, Slade SG. *Refractive Surgery.* New York: Thieme Medical Publishers, Inc.; 1999.

CHAPTER 15

The Iris-Claw Phakic Intraocular Lens

Mihai Pop

CHAPTER CONTENTS

Jan Worst originally designed the iris-claw phakic intraocular lens (IOL), and Ophtec (Boca Raton, FL) manufactures it. Many surgeons consider IOL implantation to be the safest treatment for high myopia and high hyperopia.

Specifications
- a single piece of polymethylmethacrylate
- a convex-concave optic configuration
- optic diameter: 5 or 6 mm (depending on the power of the lens that is required)
- overall diameter: 8.5 mm.
- available in 1.0-D increments (−3.0 to −23.5 D for myopia and +1 to +12 D for hyperopia)

PREOPERATIVE CONSIDERATIONS

Advantages
- lower risk for postoperative corneal ectasia, haze, and even halos compared with photorefractive keratectomy (PRK) or laser in situ keratomileusis (LASIK) (one reason for the increasing popularity of phakic IOLs)
- true reversibility of procedure
- preservation of accommodation
- better predictability of results than with PRK and LASIK for high ametropias
- higher upper limit of treatment (only −7 to −12 D for PRK), which leads to better predictability and fewer retreatments, halos, haze, and loss of BCVA
- fewer risks than with PRK or LASIK for patients with myopia higher than 10 D or hyperopia higher than 3 D (even though 60% of these patients have excellent results from the procedure)
- lower incidence of retinal detachment than with clear lensectomy, which has a non-negligible 2% risk for retinal detachment

Indications and Inclusion Criteria
- visually disabling high myopia (>−7 D) or high hyperopia (>+3 D)
- realistic patient expectations
- patient age more than 21 years (required for refractive stability)
- endothelial cell count greater than 2000 cells/mm
- anterior chamber (AC) depth greater than 3.2 mm
- pupil size smaller than 6.5 mm

Patient Examination
- Measure manifest and cycloplegic refraction.
- Evaluate best corrected visual acuity (BCVA) and uncorrected visual acuity (UCVA) using Snellen's chart.
- Evaluate near visual acuity using a Jaeger chart.
- Measure pupil size in scotopic conditions.
- Perform corneal topography.
- Perform an endothelial cell count.
- Perform biometry to determine AC depth and axial length.
- Perform gonioscopy.
- Perform a slit-lamp examination of the anterior segment and fundus of the eye.
- Test patients with amblyopia or strabismus for BCVA.
  - Inform these patients that the procedure will not improve BCVA.
  - Exclude these patients from refractive surgery unless carefully evaluated.

Patient Preparation
- Perform surgery in a standard sterile cataract operating room layout.
- Instruct the patient to remove soft contact lenses at least 2 to 3 days before the preoperative examination.
- For rigid gas-permeable contact lenses, verify the stability of the eye's topography before surgery (stability may take 4–6 weeks).
- Administer oral analgesics to the patient 15 to 30 min before surgery.
- Constrict the pupil using pilocarpine 0.2% (3 drops every 10 min).
- Administer antibiotic drops (ofloxacin 0.3%) 30 min before surgery (1 or 2 drops every 10 min).

SURGICAL CONSIDERATIONS

Absolute Contraindications
- unstable or progressive myopia or hyperopia
- glaucoma or a family history of glaucoma
- iris abnormalities
- history of uveitis
- angle closure or visible angle trauma

Relative Contraindications
- diabetic retinopathy
- autoimmune disease, Crohn's disease, or any disease causing repeated intraocular inflammation
- amblyopia or strabismus

Methods
- Drape the patient's head.
- Insert the speculum and isolate the eyelashes.
- Anesthetize the eye with two drops of topical tetracaine 1% (e.g., Cepacol, Viractin, or Pontocaine) or peribulbar lidocaine 2% without epinephrine (Xylocaine; Abbott Laboratories, Abbott Park, IL)
- Sterilize and prepare the eye using a swab stick with proviodine.
- Ensure that the pupil is constricted by injecting carbachol 0.01% (Carbastat) into the AC.
- Avoid using epinephrine, which dilates the pupil.
- Inject subconjunctival Xylocaine 2% in the superior, nasal, and temporal quadrants (helps to decrease patient discomfort while manipulating the iris).
- Use a 6-mm, three-step, scleral-limbal incision to minimize iris prolapse (may be a superior or temporal incision).
- If bleeding occurs, lightly cauterize the incision to avoid induced astigmatism.
- The paracentesis incisions differ from those made during standard surgery.
  - Make two paracentesis incisions using a 20-gauge, 1.4-mm, V-Lance knife (one incision at the 2:00 position and one at 10:00).
  - Make parallel incisions toward the 4:00 and 8:00 positions, respectively.
  - Do not direct these stab incisions radially; they must point to the future enclavation site.

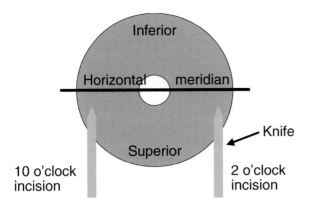

Figure 15–1 Making paracentesis incisions.

Inferior

Horizontal meridian

Superior

Knife

10 o'clock incision

2 o'clock incision

○ End the paracentesis 1 mm superior to an hypothetical horizontal meridian bisecting the pupil (Fig. 15–1).
• Inject a highly cohesive viscoelastic (sodium hyaluronate), such as Healon GV (Pharmacia, Peapack, NJ) through each paracentesis incision.
  ○ Fill the AC from the periphery toward the center.
  ○ Avoid overfilling the AC because the natural lens will bow posteriorly and the claws of the lens will bump on the inferior iris, making insertion more difficult.
• Apply viscoelastic on the lens.
• Insert the lens over the pupil through the incision using a lens-holding forcep with T-shaped lower jaw (Sinskey lens-holding forcep) with a 15-degree angle.

• Using an angled Sinskey or Kuglen hook, rotate the lens 90 degrees toward the horizontal meridian and desired position over the center of the pupil.
• Ensure that the lens is centered over the pupil.
• Use Miostat (Alcon, Forth Worth, TX) as needed to constrict the pupil.
• Visualize the iris spot where the claw will be entrapped.
• Insert the enclavation needle (provided by the manufacturer) for the claw that will be closest to the limbus. (Always insert the enclavation needle before the T-shaped forcep to hold the lens.)
• With the T-shaped, lower-jaw forcep, grasp the lens slightly toward the claw to entrap it (Fig. 15–2). (This action helps

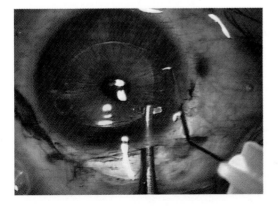

Figure 15–2 Enclavation of the lens. The T-shaped forcep holds the lens near the claw.

to avoid accidental contact with the natural lens, especially if the iris prolapses inadvertently, because the constricted iris still covers the optic and forcep.)
- Use the enclavation needle to create a small knuckle of tissue.
  ○ Begin 0.5 mm from the pinpointed spot and push forward so that the spot is at the top of the knuckle.
  ○ Insert the hook of the enclavation needle between both claws of the lens while gently lifting upward, so that the knuckle of tissue becomes entrapped by the claw.
- Perform the second iris entrapment in the same manner.
- Perform an iridectomy at the end of the surgery or after the lens is inserted if the iris tends to prolapse.
- Do not hesitate to reposition the iris-claw lens so that the lens centers on the pupil (Fig. 15–3).
- Close the incision with an "X" using nylon 10-0 suture.
- Be sure to remove all the viscoelastic before suturing. (Remaining viscoelastic may artificially push on the IOL, which could mimic a decentration and deceive the surgeon into recentering the IOL.)
- Place a protective shield on the eye, and ask the patient to wear the shield while sleeping during the first postoperative week.

Perioperative Complications
- those that occur in standard intraocular surgery
  ○ cystoid macular edema
  ○ transient corneal edema
  ○ endophthalmitis
  ○ wound leaks
- contact between the phakic IOL and natural lens during insertion (may generate a cataract postoperatively)
- iris prolapse [perform an iridectomy (Fig. 15–4)]

- angle bleeding (occurs if the IOL is slightly pulled inward while performing the second iris entrapment)
- thin iris entrapment
  ○ may cause phakic lensdonesis (see postoperative complications; Fig. 15–6)
  ○ re-enclave the lens
- decentration of the IOL (reposition the lens until centered over the pupil)
- loss of AC depth
  ○ a major complication
  ○ immediately remove the IOL

Alternative Treatments
- PRK
- LASIK
- clear lensectomy (for patients with presbyopia or mild lenticular changes)

POSTOPERATIVE CONSIDERATIONS

Medications
- Prescribe antibiotic drops (oflaxacin 0.3% and tobramycin 0.3% plus dexamethasone 0.1%) four times a day for the first month.

Results with Myopia.
- Pop et al
  ○ postoperative refraction of -0.75 ± 1.10 D
  ○ 71% of eyes within ± 1 D of emmetropia
  ○ no loss of BCVA
  ○ one or more lines of BCVA gained by 26% of eyes
  ○ mild halos or glare for 22% of eyes but no major complications
  ○ only 9% with mild cell flare at 1 month postoperatively
  ○ 26% of mild decentration of 0.25 to 0.5 mm inferior from the center of the pupil
  ○ stable refraction at 1 to 3 months postoperatively
  ○ no contact between the IOL and natural lens

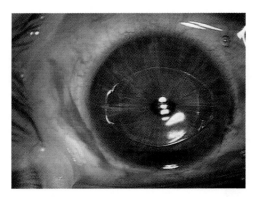

Figure 15–3 View of the iris-claw immediately after surgery.

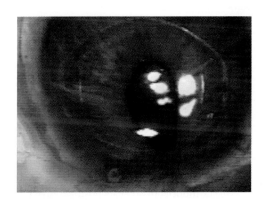

Figure 15–4 Iris prolapse during surgery.

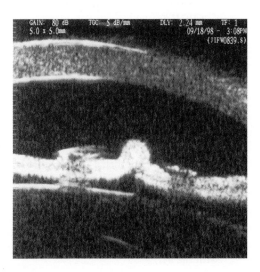

Figure 15–5 Intraocular micrograph of the iris-claw lens in the AC showing normal iris entrapment.

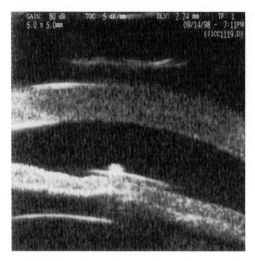

Figure 15–6 Intraocular micrograph of the iris-claw lens in the AC showing thin iris entrapment that may result in phakic lens-donesis (see Postoperative Complications).

- ○ distance between the lens and posterior surface of the IOL usually 0.78 to 0.93 mm
- ○ the pigment layer of the iris should not be disturbed by the presence of the IOL
- ○ original AC depth reduced by 28 to 34% after implantation
- Menezo et al
  - ○ postoperative spherical equivalent of −0.21 ±1.26 D
  - ○ 80% of eyes within ±1.00 D of emmetropia and 50% of eyes within 0.50 D of emmetropia
  - ○ halos in 23% of eyes (attributable to IOL optic size)
  - ○ particularly severe halos in eyes with decentration
  - ○ decentration in up to 12% of eyes
  - ○ no permanent loss of more than one line of BCVA visual acuity with the convex-concave model
  - ○ stable refraction between the first and the third postoperative month
  - ○ no cataract formation, retinal detachment, or related cases of glaucoma 2 years postoperatively
  - ○ endothelial cell loss of 8 to 17% (cell endothelial injury probably occurs during surgery but morphometric changes in the cells recover after 4 years and gradually approach preoperative levels after slight progressive cell loss after implantation)

Results with Hyperopia
- fewer data available for hyperopic iris-claw lenses (compared with myopic lenses)
- Fechner et al
  - ○ spherical equivalent of 0.03 ±1.67 D at 12 months to 10 years postoperatively
  - ○ no contact between the IOL and natural lens
  - ○ no permanent loss of more than one line of BCVA

Postoperative Complications
- halos, glare, and starburst
  - ○ Considerable halos may result if the pupil is 1 mm larger than the optic diameter.
  - ○ Choose optic diameter carefully.
- endothelial cell loss
  - ○ Perform an endothelial cell count at 6, 12, and 24 months postoperatively.
  - ○ If abnormal progressive endothelial cell loss occurs, consider removing the lens.
- pigments released from the iris onto the IOL (rare, but caused by IOL contact with the iris)

- phakic lensdonesis
  - Both claws do not entrap enough iris tissue.
  - Consider repositioning the lens because of increased risk for endothelial cell loss.
- decentration
  - Consider repositioning the IOL if the patient complains of disturbing halos or glare.
- lens dislocation
  - Reposition the lens immediately to minimize damage to the endothelium.

Enhancements and Secondary Procedures
- Verify if the surgery has increased the amount of astigmatism. (If the incisions are responsible for such an increase, wait for 6 months or for refractive stability, before considering possible enhancements.)
- For ametropia, phakic IOL implantation may be combined with PRK or LASIK.

Postoperative Care and Follow-Up
- Provide each patient with an emergency telephone number so that medical care may be provided as quickly as possible if needed.
- Examine the eye 1 day, 1 and 2 weeks, and 2, 3, 6, 12, and 24 months after surgery.
- Measure manifest refraction.
- Evaluate BCVA and UCVA using Snellen's chart.
- Perform an endothelial cell count.
- Perform corneal topography.
- Compare current data with previous data on intraocular pressure.
- Verify decentration of the lens over time.
- The AC can be examined with the ultrasound biomicroscope.

Suggested Readings

Fechner P, van der Heijde G, Worst J. The correction of myopia by lens implantation into phakic eyes. *Am J Ophthalmol.* 1989;107:659.

Fechner PU, Singh D, Wulff K. Iris-claw in phakic eyes to correct hyperopia: preliminary study. *J Cataract Refract Surg.* 1998;24:48–56.

Güel JL, Vazquez M, Gris O, De Muller A, Manero F. Combined surgery to correct high myopia: iris claw phakic intraocular lens and laser in situ keratomileusis. *J Refract Surg.* 1999;15:529–537.

Menezo JL, Avino JA, Cisneros A, Rodriguez-Salvador V, Martinez-Costa R. Iris claw intraocular lens for high myopia. *J Refract Surg.* 1997;13:545–555.

Menezo JL, Cisneros AL, Hueso JR, Harto M. Long-term results of surgical treatment of high myopia with Worst-Fechner intraocular lenses. *J Cataract Refract.* 1995;21:93–98.

Menezo JL, Cisneros AL, Rodriguez-Salvador V. Endothelial study of iris-claw phakic lens: four years follow-up. *J Cataract Refract Surg.* 1998;24:1039–1049.

Pérez-Santoja J, Bueno JL, Zato MA. Surgical correction of high myopia in phakic eyes with Worst-Fechner myopia intraocular lenses. *J Refract Surg.* 1997;13:268–284.

Pop M, Mansour M, Payette Y. Ultrasound biomicroscopy of the iris-claw phakic intraocular lens for high myopia. *J Refract Surg.* 1999;15:632–635.

Trindale F, Pereira F, Cronemberger S. Ultrasound biomicroscopic imaging of posterior chamber phakic intraocular lens. *J Refract Surg.* 1998;14:497–503.

CHAPTER 16

The Posterior-Chamber Implantable Contact Lens

Louis E. Probst and Steven L. Ziémba

CHAPTER CONTENTS

Refractive surgery for extreme ametropias (myopia > -12.00 D and hyperopia $> +4.00$ D) has progressed tremendously since around 1990, but not without drawbacks and controversy. Radial keratotomy (RK), photokeratectomy (PRK), laser in situ keratomileusis (LASIK), and phakic intraocular lens (IOL) insertion all involve certain risks that may not balance their advantages (Table 16–1). For example, anterior chamber (AC) IOLs are relatively easy to insert and produce excellent predictable refractive results, but they may put the integrity of the corneal endothelium and AC angle at risk for complications that may occur more than 40 years in the future. Table 16–2 compares IOL implantation and cataract surgery.

Advantages
- irrelevance of corneal thickness
- ability to correct a wide range of refractive errors
- better optics from refractive correction close to the nodal point of the eye

- less optical degradation
- no regression
- excellent predictability of results
- preservation of accommodation
- small astigmatically neutral incision with the foldable IOL

THE STAAR IMPLANTABLE CONTACT LENS

In 1986, Svyatoslov Fyodorov introduced a one-piece silicone IOL for use in phakic patients. Cataract formation and uveitis were early concerns, and cataract formation from his early "top hat" design was reported as late as 1993. STAAR Surgical Co. refined Fyodorov's IOL design by incorporating collagen into the IOL material, which has improved the biocompatability and results obtained with today's STAAR implantable contact lens (ICL) (STAAR model MIS-PF or MSI-TF injector and STAAR model FTP foam-tipped plunger with STAAR model SFC-45 cartridge).

TABLE 16–1

Limitations of Refractive Procedures for Extreme Ametropias

Procedure	Major Complications*	Possible Complications	Problems
PRK	Haze	Cataracts	Prolonged steroid use
LASIK	Regression	Ectasia	Insufficient corneal thickness/stability
ICL	Cataracts (1–10%) Glaucoma Pigment dispersion (4%) Pupillary block (4%)	Long-term cataracts Focal closure of AC angle	Improper sizing of ICL
Artisan iris-claw phakic IOL	Endothelial cell loss (4–5%/year) Chronic AC flare Decentrations (43%) Retinal detachment (<1%)	Cataracts Secondary glaucoma	Lens not foldable
NuVita AC phakic IOL	Pupillary ovalization (22.6%) Endothelial cell loss (1–2%/year) Glare/halos (27.8%)	Cataracts Focal closure of AC angle Secondary glaucoma	Lens not foldable
Clear lens extraction	Retinal detachment		Disruption of the vitreous/posterior capsular interface
Myopic epikeratoplasty	Poor predictability/stability		Lack of corneal lenticules
Intracorneal lenses	Instability of lens		Poor biocompatability

*Percentages indicate incidence of complications in the Zaldivar studies.

TABLE 16–2

Comparison of Cataract Surgery with ICL Surgery

Cataract Surgery	ICL Surgery
IOLs are implanted into capsular bag.	ICLs are placed in front of a normal lens.
Protection of corneal endothelium is critical.	The anterior capsule must be protected.
Removal of tissue can hide surgical errors.	Tissue damage immediately obvious.
Some refractive errors are tolerated.	Predictability of results is essential.
Speed and efficiency are emphasized.	ICL placement is a delicate procedure.

Specifications

- porcine collagen/hydroxyethylmethy-lacrylate copolymer
- refractive index of 1.45 at 35°C
- plate haptic design
- foldable
- implantable through a 3.0-mm corneal incision

- central concave/convex optic sizes [4.5–5.5 mm in diameter; a 4.8-mm optic on a posterior-chamber (PC) phakic lens is the equivalent of a 6.05-mm optical refractive zone on the cornea; e.g., for the 5.5-mm lens, its equivalent corneal optical zone is 6.9 mm]
- myopic IOLs available (−3.0 to −20.0 D)
- hyperopic IOLs available (+3.0 to +17.0 D)
- five ICL lengths are manufactured (11.0 mm, 11.5 mm, 12.0 mm, 12.5 mm, and 13.0 mm)
- rests in front of, but not on, the anterior capsule

PREOPERATIVE CONSIDERATIONS

Indications
- refractive error (extreme errors uncorrectable by LASIK because of poor predictability or inability to maintain adequate corneal thickness)
- corneal thickness insufficient for LASIK
- overcorrection from previous refractive surgeries
- keratoconus (possible correction)
- amblyopia (possible correction)

Inclusion Criteria
- stable refraction for the last 12 months
- AC depth of at least 2.8 mm
- good general health
- good ocular health
- preoperative consent with explanation of alternatives

Patient Preparation and Evaluation
- discontinuation of contact lens wear (≥ 2 weeks for soft contact lenses and ≥ 4 weeks for rigid gas-permeable lenses)
- measurement of refractive stability (must have been stable for more than 1 year) and refractive parameters
- dilated ocular examination
- manifest and cycloplegic refraction (myopic patients usually prescribed an ICL power approximately 3.0–5.0 D above the spherical portion of manifest refraction; for hyperopes, the difference is ~5.0–7.0 D)
- keratometry (preferably by corneal topography)
- measurement of AC depth (from corneal endothelium to anterior capsule)
- central pachymetry
- axial length by A-scan ultrasonography
- calculation of the appropriate ICL model and diopter based solely on biometric and refractive data
  - currently handled by STAAR Surgical Co.
  - performed with formulas developed by Feingold and Olsen
- estimation of the diameter of the ciliary sulcus (i.e., white-to-white limbal measurement) to determine the degree to which the ICL vaults in front of the crystalline lens
  - Measure the distance with calipers at least three times to ensure accuracy.
  - Perform topography using devices such as the Orbscan II (Orbtek Inc., Salt Lake City, UT) or the Vista Hand-Held Corneal Topographer (EyeSys/Premier, Jacksonville, FL)].
- choice of the proper ICL size
  - Add 0.5 mm to the white-to-white measurement for myopic lenses.
  - Subtract 0.5 mm from the white-to-white measurement for hyperopic lenses.
  - To ensure proper central vaulting of the myopic ICL, modulate the chosen lens size based on anterior chamber depth (ACD) (Table 16–3). (Accommodation of the crystalline lens primarily occurs by changes to its posterior plane and is therefore not affected by the ICL,

TABLE 16–3

Selection of the Size of the ICL

AC Depth (mm)	Amount to Add to White-to-White Measurement
<2.8	0; ICL implantation contraindicated
2.8–3.0	0; white-to-white measurement ±0.5 mm as described
3.1–3.5	0.25 mm (to maximum length of 13.0 mm)
>3.5	0.50 mm (to maximum length of 13.0 mm)

which appears to differentially vault as the lens accommodates.)

○ If these measurements suggest a lens size between the available ICL lengths, choose the next largest size if the eye has a large angle (>0.7 mm) or the next smaller size if the angle is small (<0.7 mm) (e.g., an eye with a white-to-white measurement of 11.25 mm, an ACD of 3.3 mm, and a large angle should get a 12.0-mm lens).

Peripheral Iridotomies

An iridotomy is a procedure that creates a small hole in the outer part of the iris to connect the PC and AC of the eye. This allows the aqueous fluid to drain easily to the AC.

Indications

- prophylactic prevention of the development of pupillary block glaucoma following ICL implantation

Equipment

- a neodymium:yttrium-aluminum-garnet laser
- an argon-krypton laser
- combination of both lasers

Methods

- Schedule 1 to 2 weeks before ICL implantation.
- Set laser power settings as low as possible (1–5 mW).
- Pretreat with an argon laser to reduce intraoperative bleeding.

- Minimize any damage to the underlying lens capsule by using the lowest power and the fewest laser pulses.
- Place the iridotomies at approximately the 10:00 and 2:00 positions on the peripheral iris and no more than 90 degrees (3 hr on a clock face) apart.
- Ensure that at least one iridotomy is patent after ICL placement.
- Make each iridotomy 0.8 to 1.0 mm in diameter.
- Verify patency before ICL surgery.

SURGICAL CONSIDERATIONS

Absolute Contraindications

- history or clinical signs of ocular disease
  ○ cataracts
  ○ iritis/uveitis in either eye
  ○ diabetic retinopathy in either eye
  ○ glaucoma in either eye
  ○ progressive sight-threatening disease (other than myopia)
  ○ pigmentary dispersion syndrome
  ○ pseudoexfoliation syndrome
- visually significant pre-existing lens opacities causing best corrected visual acuity (BCVA) of 20/40 or worse

Relative Contraindications

- blindness in the fellow eye (monocularity)
- unrealistic patient expectations
- irregular astigmatism
- unstable refraction
- age greater than 50 years (consider refractive lensectomy; see Chapter 13)

Equipment

- Occucoat or STAARVISC viscoelastic substance
- diamond keratome, 2.7 or 3.2 mm (model no. N03820; Diamatrix Ltd. Inc., The Woodlands, TX)
- trifacet keratome for paracentesis or any diamond blade (e.g., Diamatrix, model no. N03420)
- Lindstrom lens insertion forceps without notch (model no. SP2325; Rhein Medical Inc., Tampa, FL)
- lens tucker (model no. 6-479; Duckworth & Kent)
- Nugent (blunt) forceps (to open lens vial)
- manual or automated irrigation/aspiration (I/A) set-up

Medications

- drops for achieving maximal pupillary dilation
  - tropicamide 1% or cyclopentolate 1% (5–10 min, 3–4 times)
  - phenylephrine 2.5% (3–4 times, 5–10 min before surgery
  - flurbiprofen, 0.03% (2–3 times daily for 2 days prior to surgery to reduce miosis)

Anesthesia

- Use anesthesia as for cataract surgery.
- Although ICL implantation may be accomplished under topical or local anesthesia, new ICL surgeons should utilize local anesthesia (peribulbar or retrobulbar) to provide good prolonged akinesia and anesthesia.
- Once new surgeons have mastered the ICL implantation technique, they can perform it effectively under topical anesthesia in less than 15 min.
- topical anesthesia (one of the following)
  - proparacaine 0.5% (one drop, 5–10 min, 3–4 times)
  - lidocaine 1%–4% (one drop, 5–10 min, 3–4 times)

- Marcaine 0.5% (one drop, 5–10 min, 3–4 times)
- peribulbar local anesthesia
  - lidocaine 1% (5 cc without epinephrine)
  - $\frac{5}{8}$ inch 25-G needle
  - higher potential for globe perforation in high myopes
- retrobulbar local anesthesia
  - lidocaine 1% (5 cc without epinephrine)
  - a 1.5 inch 27-G needle
  - results in less chemosis than peribulbar approach
  - higher potential for globe perforation in high myopes

Methods

- Dilate eye as indicated above.
- Confirm a minimum dilation of 8 mm before proceeding with ICL implantation.
  - Less than 8 mm requires excessive distortion of the ICL to place it behind the iris and is thus too small for safety.
  - If the pupil will not dilate to 8 mm, abort surgery.
- Prepare and drape the ocular area as for cataract surgery.
- Lubricate the lens chamber, loading area, and barrel of the lens injector cartridge with several drops of balanced saline solution (BSS).
- Grasp the ICL with the lens-loading forceps.
- Verify the correct orientation with dimple on right leading haptic.
  - A properly oriented lens has a dimple on the leading right-hand footplate and the trailing left-hand footplate.
  - If these dimples are reversed, the lens is upside down.
  - Avoid using an upside-down lens because the lens is designed to have an anterior vault to allow its central portion to clear the crystalline lens (an upside-down lens will touch the central crystalline lens).

- Place the ICL into the loading barrel of the cartridge *before* making any incisions (so that any delays in loading do not cause delays in the middle of the surgical procedure).
- Tuck the sides of the ICL into the sidewall grooves of the cartridge.
- Lubricate with BSS.
- Place viscoelastic in front of and behind ICL to reduce bubble formation.
- Place the foam-tipped plunger in the injector pen.
- Hydrate the foam-tipped plunger with BSS.
- Retract the foam-tipped plunger into injector pen.
- Load the lens cartridge (containing the ICL) into the injector pen.
- Advance the plunger to push the ICL into view in the cartridge barrel.
- Again, verify the correct orientation of the ICL (reload if orientation is incorrect or questionable).
- Once loaded, keep the ICL and cartridge hydrated with BSS.
- Retract the plunger about 2 mm and then advance it to just behind the ICL.
- Again, check the pupil to verify that it is dilated to a minimum of 8 mm (10 mm preferred).
  - If not dilated fully, abort surgery until appropriate dilation is achieved.
  - Note: Intracameral lidocaine anesthesia may induce constriction of the pupil. If you use intracameral lidocaine, also use epinephrine diluted to 1:1,000 strength to maintain adequate mydriasis.
- Insert the lid speculum (never place surgical instruments near pupillary center).
- Make one or two paracentesis incisions 60 to 90 degrees away from the proposed area of the main incision.
- Make a beveled 3.2-mm clear corneal tunnel incision (corneal tunnel ideally 1.50–1.75 mm long).

- Place the viscoelastic cannula just inside the wound lip during injection (never insert the viscoelastic cannula across the pupil)
- Inject viscoelastic only until ripples or swirls form in the AC.
  - Do not overinflate the AC with viscoelastic (may push the iris diaphragm down onto crystalline lens making ICL positioning difficult).
  - Do not attempt to inject the viscoelastic around the zonules (may trap viscoelastic under the iris).
- Slowly inject the ICL (Fig. 16–1).
  - *Never* allow the cartridge tip to come near the pupillary center.
  - Inject the ICL with the cartridge only partially in the incision.
  - Do not inject ICL quickly.
  - Allow the leading haptic to unfold slowly after injecting 75% of the ICL.
  - Gently pulsate the injection of the rest of the ICL to encourage the ICL to unfold.
  - Do not rotate the ICL over the crystalline lens capsule.
  - Do not push on the ICL with the I/A tip.

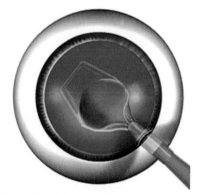

Figure 16–1 Schematic drawing depicting the insertion of the STAAR implantable contact lens (ICL).

- Never attempt to lift the iris or "massage" the ICL to resolve iris capture.
- Again, verify ICL orientation (the dimple on the right-hand leading haptic). (If the ICL is upside down, remove the ICL using the trailing footplates.)
- Place the leading footplates first under the iris.
- Lift and gently tuck the footplates and haptics under the iris.
- Constrict the pupil using acetylcholine chloride (Miochol; CIBA Vision Ophthalmics).
- Remove as much viscoelastic as possible from the AC after ICL implantation.

Intraoperative Complications
- twisting or turning of the ICL during implantation
- ICL flips upside-down when injector pen removed from incision
- ICL footplate folds
- back end of ICL sticks in small incision
- a rip in the ICL haptic

POSTOPERATIVE CONSIDERATIONS

Immediate Postoperative Care
- Administer topical medications in the recovery room.
  - pilocarpine 0.5 or 2% (one drop, 3 times over 10 min)
  - diclofenac sodium (one drop; Voltaren, Roxane; CIBA Vision Ophthalmics)
  - ofloxacin 0.3% (Ocuflox, Allergan; one drop, 4 times a day for 4 days, then 3 times a day for 4 days, then 2 times a day for 4 days, then 1 time a day for 4 days)
  - prednisolone acetate 1% (Pred-Mild, Econopred, Ocu-Pred, AK-Pred, Inflamase, Pred-Forte; one drop, 4 times a day for 4 days, then 3 times a day for 4 days, then 2 times a day for 4 days, then 1 time a day for 4 days)
- Give postoperative instructions to the patient.
- Check intraocular pressure (IOP) approximately 2 to 3 hr postoperatively and treat as necessary (Table 16–4).

Follow-Up
- days 1 and 7 and months 1, 3, 6, and 12
  - Measure IOP.
  - Measure ICL vaulting (should be ~25% of ICL thickness, but do not be concerned if the lens appears to be vaulted slightly >25% because it tends to "settle down" into the sulcus within a few days).
  - Check uncorrected visual acuity (usually excellent immediately but may improve slightly over 2–3 weeks).

TABLE 16–4
Treatment of Elevated IOP after ICL Implantation

Intraocular Pressure (mmHg)	Potential Problem	Management
<21	None	Regular 24-hr follow-up
>21 and pupil constricted	Retained viscoelastic Blocked iridotomy	IOP-reducing agents [e.g., topical beta-blockers (Betagan, Allergan)] Topical pilocarpine Release of fluid Repeat iridotomies
>40 and pupil dilated	Blocked iridotomy	Release of fluid Repeat iridotomies

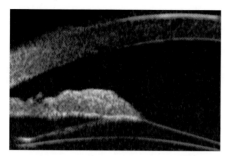

Figure 16–2 Anterior segment ultrasound 1 week after successful implantation that shows the ICL. The iris–ICL contact along the edge of the pupil is evident.

- ○ Check corrected refraction (should be stable within 1 month).
- ○ Evaluate the patency of the iridotomies.
- ○ Evaluate the clarity of the crystalline lens capsule.
- • Evaluate the position of the ICL and its interaction with structures of the anterior segment (Fig. 16–2) using ultrasound biomicroscopic imaging (essential for assessing association of findings with major complications).

- ○ ICL–iris contact
- ○ reduction in AC depth
- ○ narrowing of the AC angle opening
- ○ peripheral contact of the ICL with the crystalline lens
- • Examine the patient as needed under a standard antibiotic/anti-inflammatory regimen [e.g., patients in a U.S. clinical study received ofloxacin and tobramycin/dexamethasone (Tobradex; Alson, Surgical Fort Worth, TX) 4 times a day for 4 days tapering off over 16 days].*

Results[†]

- • excellent (when the severity of the preoperative prescription is considered)
- • a lower percentage of patients achieving 20/20 and 20/40 uncorrected vision than

*Advise the patient that the prescription for Tobradex may not be refilled because overuse may induce secondary lens opacification (i.e., cataracts).

[†]These results are from Zaldivar R (1998) (Table 16–5).

TABLE 16–5

Results of ICL Implantation for High Myopia and Hyperopia (Zaldivar)

	Myopia	Hyperopia
Number of eyes	124	24
Mean refractive error (range)	−13.4 ± 2.2 D (−8.0 to −18.6 D)	+6.5 ± 2.1 D +3.8 to +10.5 D)
Follow-up	≤ 36 months	18 months
Efficacy		
20/20	2%	8%
20/40	68%	63%
Predictability		
+/−0.5 D	44%	58%
+/−1.0 D	69%	79%
≥ 2 or more lines of visual acuity gained	36%	8%
≥ 2 or more lines of visual acuity lost	0.8%	4%

Source: Zaldivar R, Davidorf JM, Oscherow S. Posterior chamber phakic intraocular lens for myopia of −8 to −19 diopters. *J Refract Surg.* 1998;14:294–305; Davidorf JM, Zaldivar R, Oscherow S. Posterior chamber phakic interocular lens for hyperopia of +4 to +11 diopters. *J Refract Surg.* 1998;14:306–311.

what we have come to expect for LASIK (many already had a reduced BCVA preoperatively)
- improved BCVA of two or more lines (36% of the myopic group; offers extremely exciting opportunities for the improvement of the vision in this somewhat disabled group)

Complications[‡]
- pigmentary dispersion (from ICL–iris contact)
- anterior subcapsular cataract formation (from ICL–crystalline lens contact)
- pupillary block
  - IOP spikes that occur in the immediate (first 24 hr) postoperative period usually result from nonpatent iridotomies or, rarely, secondary pupillary dilation that closes off the iridotomies
  - IOP spikes at 5 to 10 days postoperatively (rarely reported as a result of retained viscoelastic that causes aqueous misdirection; emphasizes need for carefully performed iridotomies as well as evacuation of viscoelastic from the eye)
- iatrogenic cataracts
  - localized "point" opacifications [caused by surgical trauma during ICL implantation (Fig. 16–3) but usually do not progress or become sight-threatening]
  - central, nonlocalized, anterior subcapsular opacifications (reported in a few cases associated with no anterior vaulting above the central capsule and caused by a lens that was too small or was placed upside down in the eye, causing the lens to vault backward)

[‡]See Table 16–6 for more complications.

TABLE 16–6
Complications of ICL Implantation

Complication	Incidence
Pupillary block	4.8%
ICL-related IOP spike	1.6%
Steroid-induced IOP spike	4.8%
Inverted IOL	0.8%
IOL extraction	4.0%
ICL decentration	
<1 mm	14.5%
>1 mm	2.4%
Broken IOL	0.8%
Lens opacities	2.4%
Retinal detachment	0.8%
Other potential complications not reported	
ICL too small (poor vaulting)	
ICL too big (excessive vaulting)	
Pigmentary dispersion/pigmentary glaucoma	
Glare/halos	

Source: Zaldivar R, Davidorf JM, Oscherow S. Posterior chamber phakic intraocular lens for myopia of −8 to −19 diopters. *J Refract Surg.* 1998;14:294–305.

- crystalline lens opacification (estimated incidence of <1%–10%)
- late-term cataracts (reported without a direct association to surgical trauma)

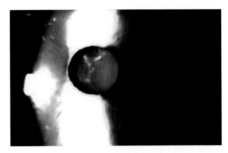

Figure 16–3 An anterior subcapsular cataract 5 weeks after ICL implantation. Uncorrected visual acuity was still 20/25.

- longer-term studies and follow-up required to evaluate their incidence and etiology
- pigmentary glaucoma
  - usually results from debridement of the anterior iris surface during lens manipulation or from surgical iridotomies (not recommended)
  - generally resolves within the first few weeks (indicates that it did not result from chafing of the posterior iris)
- glare or halos (rare except for patients with physiologically large pupils)

Treatment of Complications
- pupillary block from high IOP
  - Treat with topical antiglaucoma medications.
  - Release the aqueous fluid through the paracentesis incision.
  - Constrict the pupil with pilocarpine to open the iridotomies.
  - Repeat the laser iridotomies.
- iatrogenic cataracts
  - Remove the ICL and replace it with next larger size (recommended by STAAR if the ICL is observed with <25% anterior central vaulting at 3 months or more postoperatively to preclude anterior capsule opacification or iris chafing).
- pigmentary glaucoma (If pigment deposits are persistent and associated with elevated IOP, consider removing the ICL.)
  - Maximally dilate the pupil.
  - Inject viscoelastic at the edge of the ICL to elevate it above the capsule.
  - Grasp one of the footplates with forceps.
  - Pull the ICL above the iris.
  - Pull the ICL through a 3.0-mm incision without folding or cutting it.
  - Insert a new ICL as described (see pp. 172–174).

INTRAOCULAR LENS INSERTION AND LASER IN SITU KERATOMILEUSIS (BIOPTICS)

The ultimate goal of the refractive surgeon is the correction of any refractive error. ICLs allow surgeons to correct a wide range of spherical refractive errors, but many of these eyes also have large amounts of astigmatism. Roberto Zaldivar, MD, conceived the concept of "bioptics" to allow for full correction of virtually any refractive error.

Indications
- the correction of large refractive errors and the elimination of low to moderate levels of myopia and astigmatism (using the precision and predictability of LASIK)

Methods
- Perform the peripheral iridotomies.
- Correct the spherical component of the refractive error by implanting the ICL.
- One month later, after achieving refractive stability, correct the residual spherical and astigmatic components with LASIK (Fig. 16–4).

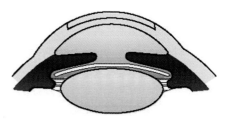

Figure 16–4 A schematic of the bioptics concept, which utilizes the ICL and LASIK to correct large spherical and astigmatic refractive errors.

Suggested Readings

Davidorf JM, Zaldivar R, Oscherow S. Posterior chamber phakic intraocular lens for hyperopia of +4.0 to +11 diopters. *J Refract Surg.* 1998;14:306–311.

Rosen E, Gore C. STAAR collamer posterior chamber phakic intraocular lens to correct myopia and hyperopia. *J Cataract Refract Surg.* 1998;24:596–606.

Trindade F, Pereira F. Cataract formation after posterior chamber phakic intraocular lens implantation. *J Cataract Refract Surg.* 1998;24: 1661–1663.

Trindade F, Pereira F, Cronemberger S. Ultrasound biomicroscopic imaging of posterior chamber phakic intraocular lens. *J Refract Surg.* 1998;14:497–503.

Zaldivar R, Davidorf JM, Oscherow S. Phakic intraocular lenses. In: Buratto L, Brint S, ed. *LASIK.* Thorofare, NJ: Slack Inc.; 1998.

Zaldivar R, Davidorf JM, Oscherow S. Posterior chamber phakic intraocular lens for myopia of −8 to −19 diopters. *J Refract Surg.* 1998;14: 294–305.

CHAPTER 17

Experience with the IVI Medennium Phakic Intraocular Lens

Kenneth J. Hoffer and Dimitrii D. Dementiev

CHAPTER CONTENTS

THE POSTERIOR CHAMBER PHAKIC LENS

The concept of a purely posterior chamber (PC) phakic refractive lens (PRL) originated in the former Soviet Union. The first PRL consisted of a completely new nontoxic silicone material that had a higher refractive index than the previous *Mushroom* model (named after its mushroom shape visible on cross section) and was completely different in its configuration, parameters, and mechanism of fixation (the *Mushroom* model was

pupil fixated; Fig. 17–1). This lens was the prototype of all other PC PRLs that are available today (Fig. 17–2).

Specifications
- intended for implantation in the PC laying on the zonular fibers
- optical zone (OZ) diameter = 5.0 mm
- total length = 11.3 mm

Advantages
- safety
- predictable results

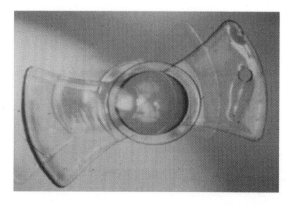

Figure 17–1 An example of the *Mushroom* model.

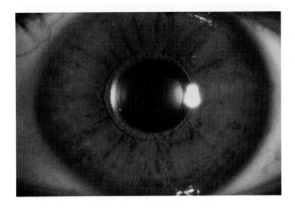

Figure 17–2 First model PRL with pupillary capture.

• reversibility of procedure
• not expensive for the doctor or patient
• helps to achieve immediate and stable refractive effect
• helps to increase uncorrected visual acuity (UCVA) and best corrected visual acuity (BCVA)

Indications
• high myopia (≥ -10.0 D)

The IVI MEDENNIUM Phakic Refractive Lens

IVI Medennium, Inc. (originally in Cincinnati, OH, but now in Irvine, CA), produces the PC PRL that we have been using for the past 6 years. A U.S. Federal Drug Administration study application is now in progress. We have implanted 483 Medennium lenses (three generations) since 1987 (Table 17–1).

TABLE 17–1

Number of Implants per Generation of Medennium PRLs

Generation	No. of Implants	Years of Use
I	97	1987–1990
II	224	Since 1990
III	162	Since 1996

Specifications
• made of silicone
• refractive index = 1.46
• OZ diameter = 4.5 to 5.5 mm (depends on the optic power of the lens)
• soft, elastic, and hydrophobic

Advantanges
• implantation easy through a 3.0- to 3.5-mm clear corneal incision
• no contact between lens and anterior capsule of the crystalline lens
• easy removal if necessary

Indications
• hyperopia (+3.0 to +15.0 D but correction possible for $\leq$ +23.0 D)
• myopia (−3.0 to −24.0 D)

Complications
• no synechiae at long-term follow-up
• decentration in the earlier, smaller models (most common complication but not observed after changing the size parameters of the PRL in successive generations)
• cataract formation
• pigmentary glaucoma (potential, not seen)

ANALYSIS OF CLINICAL DATA

The remainder of this chapter discusses our experience with second- and third-genera-

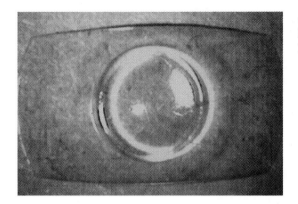

Figure 17–3 Overall design of the latest model of the silicone Russian PRL.

tion IVI Medennium PRLs (Fig. 17–3). Here we analyze clinical data for 122 implants in 72 patients (aged 9–53 years), which were collected in our day-hospitals in Milano and Bari, Italy, since 1994.

Preoperative Considerations
Inclusion Criteria
- myopia (110 cases; Table 17–2)
  - −6.00 to −23.00 D (present treatable errors)
  - −4.00 to −25.00 D (future treatable errors)
- hyperopia (12 cases; see Table 17–2)
  - +3.00 to +16.00 D (+16.00 D maximum)
  - safer to limit to +11.00 D [unless there is a deep anterior chamber (AC)

because the AC of hyperopic patients is usually shallow]
- unilateral high myopia with amblyopia in children (7 cases; see Pediatric Usage)
  - patient age 11 to 14 years
  - scleral reinforcement surgery recommended for progressive myopia
- combined astigmatism (13 cases)
  - more than 3.75 D [if >1.00 D, PRL implantation followed by additional astigmatic keratectomy (AK) no sooner than 1 month later]
- keratoconus with a high myopic component (1 case)
- refractive errors (2 cases) from radial keratectomy (RK), photorefractive keratotomy (PRK), and laser in situ keratomileusis (LASIK)

TABLE 17–2

Preoperative Refraction in Study Population

Preoperative Refraction	Percent of Total Study Population
Myopic patients (110 cases)	
−5.0 to −7.0 D	16
−7.0 D to −10.0 D	37
>−10.D	47
Hyperopic patients (12 cases)	
+3.5 to +5.0 D	67
+5.0 to + 8.0	22
>+8.0 D	11

- replacement of earlier model of the PRL (2 cases of dislocation)

Exclusion Criteria
- a clouded or nontransparent cornea
- cataracts
- lens subluxation
- glaucoma or ocular hypertension
- a shallow AC (<2.7 mm)
- vitreo/retinal problems that preclude good vision or require posterior segment intervention
- previous ocular surgery (e.g., vitreo/retinal surgery or glaucoma filtration)
- patient age more than 60 years
- diabetic retinopathy

POWER CALCULATION Accurate measurement of the precise refraction of the eye, axial length, and corneal power are imperative for proper use of the various methods of calculation.

The Russian Method: Vertex Chart
- Use the spherical equivalent of the most accurate refraction of the eye to interpolate the power of the IVI Medennium PC PRL.
- These powers are based on a simple vertex correction from 12 mm to the corneal plane.
- Although this method does not make intuitive sense optically, our experience to date shows it to be remarkably accurate.

The Holladay Refraction Formula
- Jack Holladay published a formula in the *American Journal of Ophthalmology* in 1993 for calculating the power of an intraocular lens (IOL) for an aphakic eye, ametropic pseudophakic eye (piggyback IOL), or PRL for a phakic eye.
- This method does not require measurement of the axial length but does need the corneal power, preoperative refractive error, desired postoperative refractive error, and the vertex distance of both.

- To obtain emmetropia, the formula is:

$$\text{PRL} = 1336/[(1336/\{10^3/[(10^3/R_{PRE}) - V]\} + K)] - \text{ELP} - 1336/[(1336/K) - \text{ELP}]$$

where R_{PRE} = preoperative prescription; V = vertex of R_{PRE}; K = average K; and ELP = estimated AC depth of PRL.
- To obtain ametropia, the formula is more complex:

$$\text{PRL} = 1336/[(1336/\{10^3/[(10^3/R_{PRE}) - V]\} + K)] - \text{ELP} - 1336/[(1336/\{10^3/[(10^3/R_{PO}) - V]\}+K)] - \text{ELP}$$

where R_{PO} = desired postoperative prescription; V = vertex of R_{PO}.

Medications
- Begin instillation of antibiotics drop [Tobradex (Alcon, Fort Worth, TX)] after removing contact lenses 36 to 24 hr before surgery.

Surgical Considerations
Iridectomy
- Perform a surgical or YAG iridectomy.
- surgical iridectomy at the same time as PRL implantation
  ○ Perform the basal iridectomy at the 12:00 position on the eye.
  ○ Perform the procedure after inserting the PRL.
  ○ You *must* perform a complete iridectomy. (Carefully check that the pigment layer has been cut through, ensuring that the crystalline lens has not been damaged.)
- laser iridectomy prior to PRL implantation
  ○ Perform two iridectomies with an yttrium-aluminum-garnet (YAG) laser about 2 weeks before PRL implantation at 11:00 and 1:00 on the eye.

- Avoid making the iridectomies too large.
- Make the iridectomies as peripheral as possible because light and additional images pass through them.
- One of our patients complained about night glare. (The iridectomy was large and located near the pupil edge; we sutured it and patient complaints decreased.)

Medications
- We recommend balanced saline solution (BSS) for irrigation.
- Use low-density viscoelastic.
- Administer 25 mg of oral acetazolamide 30 min before surgery.
- Mydriatics facilitate maximum pupil dilatation during surgery.
  - We *never* use atropine because the pupil needs to constrict rapidly immediately after surgery.
  - We use phenylephrine and cyclopentolate.
- The miotic acetylcholine in the AC aids pupil constriction after insertion.
- Inject corticosteroid subconjunctivally and 4.0 mg of cortisone intramuscularly at the end of the procedure (optional).
- Instill topical pilocarpine (at the end of surgery).
- Instill antibiotic drops (at the end of surgery).

Anesthesia
- Retrobulbar or peribulbar anesthesia was used exclusively and is now especially recommended.
- Topical anesthesia is not recommended.
  - It is very important that the eye not move at all during the sensitive period of haptic placement behind the iris using the spatula.
  - Sudden unexpected movement of the eye may result in damage to the crystalline lens and cause a cataract.

Instrumentation
- a clear cornea incision blade (diamond or stainless steel; 3.0–3.2 mm)
- wide Dementiev forceps (for PRL implantation; Janach Co., Italy)
- Dementiev PRO spatula-manipulator (Janach Co.)
- standard set of iris scissors and iris forceps (for manual iridectomy)
- standard lid speculum
- eye fixation forceps
- fine forceps

Methods
- handling the implant
  - After opening the sterile plastic container that holds the PRL, pick up the PRL using the special forceps.
  - Ensure that the lens does not touch the skin, conjunctiva, lids, lashes, or epithelium of the cornea because certain microelements are attracted to and become deposited on the lens surface.
  - Grasp the implant with the forceps in the correct position (longitudinal).
  - Verify positioning by ensuring that the anterior surface of the lens is up and the posterior surface is down.
  - The PRL has a similar convexity (curvature) that parallels that of a natural lens.
  - Do not squeeze the PRL too hard because it is easily damaged.
  - Do not fold the lens because it folds itself during insertion.
  - After confirmation of correct grasping and orientation of the PRL in the forceps, irrigate profusely with BSS in a syringe.
  - Inspect the PRL carefully.
  - Remove any foreign particulate matter or fibers that may have become attached to its surface with fine forceps.
  - The PRL is now ready for insertion.

- making the incision
  - Do *not* begin surgery if the diameter of the pupil is less than 5.0 mm.
  - Usually place the incision at the temporal cornea.
  - Our experience recommends performing a clear corneal, self-sealing incision 3.0 to 3.2 mm wide.
  - Use a type of incision for self-sealing cataract surgery that allows nonsutured closure of the wound.
  - Use a diamond or stainless-steel blade to make the incision.
  - Use any method of fixation to ensure that the blade does not contact the anterior lens capsule (pupil is widely dilated).
- viscoelastic insertion
  - Immediately fill the AC with viscoelastic substance to achieve a chamber at least 3.0 mm deep.
  - Also place some viscoelastic under the iris to make more room for lens insertion in the PC.
- paracentesis
  - Create an additional entry point for the lens manipulator that facilitates positioning of the PRL in the PC.
  - Make this incision with a stainless-steel or diamond knife.
  - We create an incision no larger than 1.0 to 1.5 mm and place it at the 12:00 position.
  - Hold the knife perpendicular to the corneal surface.
  - Make the cut at the limbus, so that the iridectomy is more basal so light does not pass through the iridectomy, the upper lid covers the iridectomy (fewer halos), and the iridectomy does not become blocked by the edge of the PRL (pupillary block).
- lens insertion
  - *This is the most important and delicate step of the procedure.*
  - Do *not* (1) damage the implant because it is very soft, thin, and rather expensive (Fig. 17–4), (2) damage the anterior capsule with the forceps, or (3) touch the endothelium with the implant or forceps.
  - Grasp the implant with the special forceps that are designed to protect the OZ of the PRL (only the haptic area of the implant touches the forceps).
  - Insert the PRL through a 3.0- to 3.2-mm incision without any additional folding.
  - After inserting the implant into the AC, gently open the forceps to release the lens.
  - The eye must make no unexpected sudden movements during this crucial maneuver.
  - If the PRL is upside down, it is necessary to remove it.
- retro-iris placement and centration
  - Manipulate the peripheral edges of the PRL under the iris.
  - Using the spatula-PRL manipulator (entered from the paracentesis at 12:00), move the two lateral edges of the lens under the pupil margin and under the iris.
  - Pay maximum attention to the amount of pressure that you exert on the crystalline lens capsule (too much pressure will damage the anterior capsule and cortex).
  - Try to fold the PRL with the spatula and then release it under the iris to avoid damage to the zonular fibers.
  - When all four "feet" are satisfactorily under the iris, gently center the PRL OZ using the spatula-PRL manipulator (Fig. 17–5).
- iridectomy
  - We recommend injecting acetylcholine solution into the AC to constrict the pupil as much as possible before performing the iridectomy.
  - We prefer to perform the iridectomy at 12:00 through the paracentesis site.

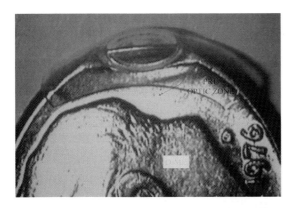

Figure 17–4 Example of the size and thickness of the silicone PRL compared with a dime.

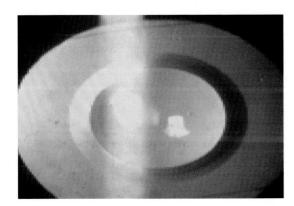

Figure 17–5 IVI-Medennium PRL well-centered in the PC with 20/20 UCVA.

○ Make the iridectomy as peripheral as possible to decrease the risk of blockage by the PRL.

○ If bleeding occurs during this step, we prefer to reinject viscoelastic as a tamponade in the area of bleeding.

○ After an appropriate waiting period (and clotting has occurred), remove the viscoelastic.

• viscoelastic removal

○ Try to remove all the viscoelastic by irrigation with BSS.

○ If you are unable to remove all the viscoelastic, remove as much as possible and do not leave any in the AC or PC.

○ Viscoelastic in the AC or PC may lead to (1) a postoperative increase in IOP or (2) viscoelastic crystallization between the anterior capsule and the posterior surface of the implant.

○ You may use irrigation/aspiration if irrigation alone does not remove enough of the viscoelastic, but do not damage the endothelial cells.

• Suturing the incision is unnecessary.

• At the conclusion of the procedure, we prefer to inject cortisone solution subconjunctivally at 12:00 and feel it helps to close the paracentesis by the conjunctiva.

• Placing a patch on the eye is not obligatory.

Operative Complications
- damage to the PRL
  - may occur during insertion into the AC if you do not use special forceps
  - may also happen during release and manipulation of the PRL under the iris
- bleeding
  - uncommon
  - may occur during the manual surgical iridectomy
- iris damage
- lens damage
  - the worst complication possible during the actual procedure
  - possible at many points in surgery: (1) during corneal incisions because of sudden knife insertion or eyeball movement; (2) during paracentesis because of insufficient viscoelastic in the AC, too quick blade movement, or eyeball movement; (3) during implant insertion because of contact between the forceps and the anterior capsule of the lens; (4) during implant manipulation because of pushing the implant on the lens; and (5) during viscoelastic removal because of inadvertent movement of irrigation or aspiration needle or excessively forceful BSS irrigation
  - remedy with phacoemulsification with IOL implantation
- endothelial cell damage
  - from inadequate viscoelastic protection
  - from silicone in the PRL (no published data)
  - endothelium damage not noticed even when edge of PRL touches the endothelium (personal experience) perhaps because of the high endothelial cell density in younger patients
- zonular fiber damage
  - necessary to remember that a large number of zonular fibers stretch across the anterior periphery of the lens capsule

- may result from pushing the implant too strenuously under the iris
- may lead to implant dislocation and OZ decentration

Postoperative Considerations
Medications
- cortisone and antibiotic drops (Tobradex) 5 to 6 times a day for 7 to 10 days
- mydriatic drops 3 to 4 times a day for 3 days (do *not* use atropine) with 3 to 4 hr action (not complete pupil dilation)
- Diamox tablets (250 mg) twice a day on the first postoperative day and then 125 mg twice a day for 2 to 3 days
  - You may notice a transitory increase in IOP the first postoperative day, which means that viscoelastic was not completely removed from the AC or PC.
  - If the IOP is more then 20 mmHg, increase the dosage of Diamox to 250 mg, 3 to 4 times a day until the IOP is normalized.
- nonsteroid drops [10–12 days after finishing Tobradex; we use Voltaren (CIBA Vision, Atlanta, GA) for 7 days]

Complications (Table 17–3)
- increase in IOP (>30 mmHg) on first or second day postoperatively
  - The patient feels pain in the eye and complains of vision loss or headache in the temple.
  - On slit-lamp examination the chamber may be shallow, the pupil doesn't react to light or is sluggish, residual viscoelastic is in the AC or PC, and the gap between the PRL and anterior capsule is larger than normal.
  - Check the patency of the iridectomy by testing the visual and red reflex.
  - Make the iridectomy bigger or create an additional one (perhaps with a YAG laser) if it is small or closed.

TABLE 17–3

Adverse Events and Complications

Adverse Event	No. of Occurrences	% Incidence (n/N; N = 122)	Implant Generation
Corneal edema after 1 month	0	0.00	
Hyphema	0	0.00	
Macular edema	0	0.00	
Raised IOP requiring treatment ≤ 1 month postoperatively	4	3.28	II and III
Persistent raised IOP	0	0.00	
Pupillary block	1	0.82	II
Retinal detachment	0	0.00	
Cataract	1	0.82	
Nonspecific inflammatory reaction	3	2.45	II
Implant decentration[1]	4	3.27	II
Endophthalmitis	0	0.00	
Iridocyclitis	3	2.45	

[1] Implant decentration occurred in four eyes of three patients who underwent implantation with negative-power generation II lenses; one patient had implant decentration of both operated eyes. All four decentered lenses were exchanged for the generation III implant, which was designed to improve centration and avoid decentration of its OZ.

○ Reabsorb the residual viscoelastic in the chamber by administering Diamox (≤ 1.0 g/day) and keeping the pupil dilated.

○ Administer beta-blocker drops until the IOP is normalized.

○ We have witnessed four cases of increased IOP (21–27 mmHg) at the 1-week postoperative visit.

○ All four cases were treated topically with timolol maleate 0.5% ophthalmic drops and Diamox.

○ Two weeks postoperatively, the IOP was within normal limits (≤ 17 mmHg) for all four cases.

○ Pupillary block was observed in one eye 3 weeks after insertion of a second generation lens.

○ We surgically enlarged the iridectomy, which relieved the pupillary block.

○ We observed no recurrence of pupillary block.

○ Be ready to convert the procedure to phacoemulsification for crystalline lens extraction with IOL implantation.

○ Keep an IOL ready in the OR with all IOL power calculations done in advance.

• subcapsular opacity

○ To date, we have seen only one case of subcapsular opacity 13 months after surgery.

○ The patient lost one line of BCVA and has poor contrast sensitivity.

• iridocyclitis (in the near postoperative period)

○ The etiology of this complication remains unknown, but all cases occurred in hyperopic eyes with lenses produced outside the United States approximately 1 to 2 months after surgery.

○ A nonsmooth surface may have irritated the posterior surface of the iris and started the mechanism of sterile inflammation.

- This rare complication is more common in hyperopic eyes (3 cases).
- Patient complains that vision is deteriorating but there is no pain.
- On slit-lamp examination, you will notice flare and cells in the AC, some synechiae between the PRL and the pupil, and a pupil that is small and difficult to dilate.
- Combination therapy is needed: steroids, atropine, adrenaline subconjunctival injection, systemic steroids, and maximum mydriasis.
- We have had three cases of iridocyclitis, two of which occurred in the same patient who had both eyes implanted.
- Using the combination therapy noted above, we achieved a normal result within 2 to 3 days.
- We consider this type of reaction to be sterile iridocyclitis with low pigment dispersion.
- We did not exchange implants in these three cases.
- No further reactions or cataracts have formed to date.

Results

- Postoperative refractive results have not changed substantially since the earliest days after surgery (Table 17–4).
- For patients with preoperative astigmatism, we performed AK at least 1 month after PRL insertion.
- In 66.1% of cases, we obtained emmetropia.
- In 26.8% we saw a residual undercorrection (myopia) no greater than −1.00 D.
- 7.1% needed additional spectacle correction (> −1.0 but < −2.5 D; in all 6 cases the goal was to leave some residual myopia because all were presbyopic patients).
- In 46.6% of the eyes we achieved no loss of any lines of BCVA.

TABLE 17–4
Key Safety and Efficacy Variables at Last Postoperative Visit

	n/*N* (*N* = 122)	% of Population
UCVA		
20/40 or better	112	91.8
20/50 to 20/80	7	5.75
20/100 to 20/150	2	1.6
20/200	1	0.8
Lines of BCVA gained or lost		
Gained 5–7 lines	6	4.9
Gained 3–4 lines	11	9.0
Gained 2 lines	12	9.8
Gained 1 line	37	30.3
No change	52	42.6
Lost 1 line	4	3.3
Manifest sphere (compared with emmetropia)		
Within 0.0 D	39	66.1
Within ±0.5 D	8	13.6
Within ±1.0 D	6	10.2
Within ±2.0 D	4	6.8
>2.0 D	2	3.4

- In 54% we noted an increase in lines of BCVA.
- In 3.3% one line of BCVA was lost.
- Postoperative UCVA was better than preoperative BCVA in 55.1% (66/122) of the cases.
- No eyes had UCVA worse than 20/200 at the last postoperative visit.
- In eyes that required PRL exchange because of dislocation [2 of the 26 exchanges performed to date are included in this study], we achieved the same BCVA as before the first PRL insertion (Fig. 17–6).
- Average endothelial cell loss (including patients who underwent two PRL procedures) was 5%, which does not differ from that reported with cataract surgery.

Pediatric Usage

MYOPIA PRL insertion is an alternative to amblyopia treatment with aniseikonic spectacles or forced use of contact lenses. Without treatment, these eyes are destined for lifetime strabismus with deep amblyopia.

Indications

- high unilateral myopia (The youngest patient in whom we have implanted a myopic PRL was 7 years old with −14.00 D and amblyopia of 20/100 BCVA).

Advantages

- correction of myopia
- treatment of amblyopia
- prevention of strabismus
- exchangability of PRL if the refractive error changes when the child grows to adulthood
- ability to repeat the implantation if necessary

Patient Preparation

- We prefer and recommend performing scleral reinforcing surgery 1 to 2 months before implantation to slow growth of the eyeball.

Results

- 20/40 UCVA at 20 months postoperatively from 20/100 preoperatively
- all had improved BCVA 6 months postoperatively after occlusion therapy

HYPEROPIA We plan to start correcting hyperopia in the near future but currently do not have any clinical experience correcting hyperopia with PRL implantation in children.

Methods

- The surgical technique is the same as that for our adult patients except for the following.
  ○ We recommend general anesthesia.

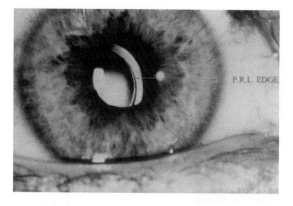

Figure 17–6 Temporal dislocation of a PC silicone PRL.

○ We also prefer manual iridectomy instead of laser iridectomy at the time of surgery.

CONCLUSION

The goal of any refractive procedure is emmetropia, and the predictability of PRL implantation provides promise for achieving it. The refractive effect may be compared with contact lenses. Reversibility is PRL implantation's most attractive feature because few refractive procedures currently may be reversed. Any skilled cataract surgeon is able to perform PRL insertion safely and easily. The complications that we have seen are not serious and were easily treated. Two main problems and complications that we need to investigate in longer follow-up are subcapsular opacities (so far we have seen only one) and pigment dispersion, which may cause glaucoma. Our study shows no pigment dispersion in negative power silicon PRLs but some slow dispersion in positive power PRLs. The ultrasound biomicroscope study showed us that the implant does not touch the anterior capsule, but we need to know more about the touching of the capsule and iris.

FUTURE APPLICATIONS

Piggyback over Intraocular Lenses

When two IOLs are necessary, it is certainly conceivable that the second lens could be a PC PRL easily inserted in the capsular bag or the ciliary sulcus. In special eyes that require piggyback lenses, the calculations of IOL power are often not as accurate and it may be necessary to exchange the more anterior lens. A PRL is much easier to remove and replace than an IOL (Fig. 17–7).

Pseudophakic Ametropia Correction

Every patient who is unhappy with the refractive results of cataract or IOL surgery could be offered a rather simple procedure of PC PRL implantation over the IOL. This application would open a whole new market for the anterior segment surgeon and replace the dangers inherent in removing and replacing a well-placed IOL in the capsular bag. Patients would more likely obtain a desirable refractive result.

Patients who wish to try monovision could have the nondominant eye implanted with an additional plus power PRL over the emmetropic IOL. If monovision was intolerable, the PRL could be easily and atraumatically slipped out.

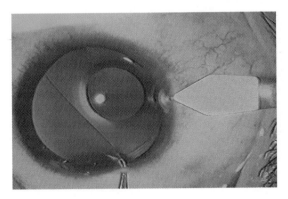

Figure 17–7 The beginning of surgery to exchange the PRL of Figure 17–6 with one that has a larger sulcus-to-sulcus diameter.

REFRACTIVE SURGERY: A COLOR SYNOPSIS

Multifocal Correction

Patients could have an emmetropic IOL implanted with a multifocal PRL placed on top of it during cataract removal. After sufficient time has passed and the patient has become accustomed to it, the patient could decide to keep the PRL or have it easily slipped out.

Patients could have a multifocal PRL placed on top of an IOL to try it out. Again, if they didn't like it, it is easily removed. Perhaps any over- or under-correction in the original IOL could also be taken into account when calculating the PRL distance power.

Suggested Readings

Asseto V, Benedetti S, Pesando P. Collamer intraocular contact lens to correct high myopia. *J Cataract Refract Surg.* 1996;22:551–556.

Baikoff G. Anterior chamber phakic IOLs. AAO Annual Meeting: 1998; New Orleans.

Baikoff G, Joly P. Comparison of minus power anterior chamber intraocular lenses and myopic epikeratoplasty in phakic eyes. *Refract Corneal Surg.* 1990;6:252–260.

Baikoff G, Arne JL, Bokobza Y, et al. Angle fixated anterior chamber lens for myopia of −7.0 to −19.0 diopters. *J Cataract Refract Surg.* 1998;14:282–293.

Chatterjee A, Shah S. Predictability of spherical PRK based on initial refraction. *J Refract Surg.* 1998;14(suppl).

Fechner PU. Intraocular lenses for the correction of myopia in phakic eyes: short term success and long term caution. *Refract Corneal Surg.* 1990;6:242–244.

Gelender H. Corneal endothelial cell loss, cystoid macular edema, and iris-supported intraocular lenses. *Ophthalmology.* 1984;91:841–846.

Hodkin M, Lemos MM, McDonald MB, Holladay JT, Shhidi SH. Near vision sensitivity after photorefractive keratectomy. *J Cataract Refract Surg.* 1997;23:2.

Holladay JT. Refractive power calculation for intraocular lenses in the phakic eye. *Am J Ophthalmol.* 1993;116:63–66.

Marinho A, Neves MC, Pinto MC, Vaz F. Posterior chamber silicone phakic intraocular lens. *J Refract Surg.* 1997;13:219–222.

CHAPTER 18

Intacs Corneal Ring Segments

Penny A. Asbell and Debby K. Holmes-Higgin

CHAPTER CONTENTS

Myopia, or nearsightedness, is the most common refractive problem in the United States; more than one fourth of the population (~70 million people) use corrective eyewear for myopia. With recent technological advances, consumers have increased interest in, as well as heightened expectations for, refractive surgery as a reasonable and viable alternative to eyeglasses and contact lenses. INTACS (KeraVision, Inc., Fremont, CA) is the third generation of the original 360-degree intrastromal corneal ring (ICR) (KeraVision, Inc.) that comprised two 150-degree arcs (Fig. 18–1).]

HISTORY

A. E. Reynolds conceived of the ring (based on expansion and contraction) in 1978; Kera Associates was formed in 1980 to develop the ring and other concepts. In 1985, the first preclinical studies of Reynolds's concept led to development of lens thickness as the means of achieving correction (as opposed to the expansion/contraction model), and in 1986, Kera-

Vision, Inc., was founded to focus solely on development of its ICR technology.

Researchers first placed the ring in animal eyes in 1985 and subsequently conducted extensive feasibility studies on various animals, including rabbits, cats, and three primate species. The rabbit became the safety model because rabbits' eyes had been used historically for ophthalmic research and safety testing (its response to a foreign body approximates that of the

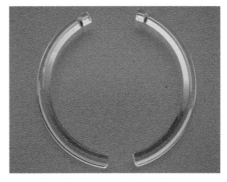

Figure 18–1 Appearance of Intacs segment before implantation.

human eye). However, no animal model had a cornea with the same thickness and morphological characteristics as the human cornea. Despite the thinness of rabbit cornea and the absence of a Bowman's membrane, researchers did not identify a more representative animal model. To refine the procedure for evaluating the ICR in live eyes, researchers inserted ICRs into the eyes of approximately 200 rabbits.

In 1991, to demonstrate the safety of the ICR in humans, researchers conducted a blind-eye trial in Brazil and a similar one in the United States shortly thereafter. Both studies demonstrated that the ICR could be safely inserted into the peripheral corneal stroma in humans, thereby flattening the central cornea; five-year follow-up demonstrated that the eye tolerated the ring well, even years after insertion. The first procedures on sighted human eyes were performed in Brazil in 1991 and in the United States in 1993 as part of a phase II study regulated by the U.S. Food and Drug Administration (FDA).

In 1995, KeraVision created intrastromal corneal ring segments (ICRS), an alternative design, and introduced them into clinical trials in the United States. A U.S. phase II study and a two-site European study were initiated in 1995. U.S. phase III (10 reporting sites) research was initiated in 1996. In April 1999, the FDA approved three sizes (0.25, 0.30, and 0.35 mm) of Intacs, the commercial name for ICRS. Intacs completely replaced the 360-degree ICR. Use of Intacs has eliminated incision-related healing complications that were noted with the 360-degree ICR. Surgeons have performed approximately 1,800 Intacs procedures clinically worldwide to date. As a nonlaser alternative that does not remove tissue from the central optical zone (OZ) and is both removable and replaceable, Intacs represent a new direction for refractive surgery.

Specifications
• two half-rings placed through a single, peripheral incision
• made of polymethylmethacrylate
• varying the thickness of Intacs changes corneal curvature and dioptric correction (a nearly linear relationship between the degree of flattening achieved and the device thickness)

Advantages
• reshaping of the cornea's anterior curvature without invading the patient's central visual axis (Fig. 18–2)
• maintenance-free correction
• rapid, predictable, and stable results
• minimal risk of loss of best corrected visual acuity (BCVA) (in FDA clinical trials that did not allow secondary interventions, 90% of patients with one implanted eye

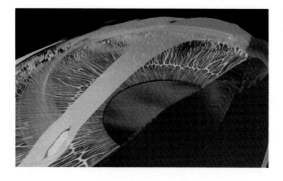

Figure 18–2 Schematic drawing of a cornea demonstrating the position of Intacs in the cornea after placement.

were very satisfied with their surgical outcome, and 95% of patients with bilateral surgery were satisfied)
- approximately 20% of patients with BCVA of 20/16 or better after primary procedures involving Intacs without enhancements (data from an FDA study)
- simple outpatient procedure performed under topical anesthesia, with little risk of incision-related complications
- preservation of tissue in central OZ
- maintenance of prolate corneal asphericity
- simple removability or replaceability (unique to Intacs and especially appealing to conservative or cautious patients)
- following removal, return of refraction to preoperative level, in most cases (according to recent data)
- excellent safety results (1.1% incidence of complications in U.S. trials)

PREOPERATIVE CONSIDERATIONS

Indications and Inclusion Criteria
- reduction or elimination of mild myopia (-1.00 to -3.00 D spherical equivalent at the spectacle plane)
- age of 21 years or older
- documented stability of refraction, as demonstrated by less than 0.50 D of change for at least 12 months prior to the preoperative examination
- $+1.00$ D or less of astigmatism

Patient Education
- Assist the patient in choosing the best procedure for his or her refractive error.
- Advise patient of realistic visual expectations and potential postoperative visual problems, including the fact that the patient may not be totally independent of spectacle lenses, as a result of this or any other refractive procedure.

- Discuss the specific advantages, limitations, and potential complications of the selected refractive procedure at an early consultation (this can save time in the long run).
- Address patient's concerns about permanently altering the eyes and the availability of options in the event that the patient is dissatisfied with the outcome.
- Discuss all known general surgical risks with patient.

Patient Preparation
- As with any surgical procedure, take precautions to minimize the risk of infection.
- Instruct the patient to discontinue application of eye makeup for 2 to 3 days before the procedure.
- Advise the patient to instill one drop of trimethoprim (Polytrim; Allergan, Inc., Irvine, CA) in the operative eye at bedtime on the night prior to the procedure.
- Instruct the patient to instill one drop of Polytrim every hour (a total of three applications) beginning 3 hr before the procedure.
- Ensure that the patient completes all administrative forms, including the patient consent form.

Preoperative Medications
- Valium (5–10 mg, 20–30 min before procedure)
- diclofenac sodium (Voltaren Ophthalmic; CIBA Vision, Atlanta, GA) drops (20–30 min prior to procedure)
- tetracaine (Cetacaine or Pontocain; apply drops upon entering operative suite)

SURGICAL CONSIDERATIONS

Absolute Contraindications
- collagen vascular, autoimmune, or immunodeficiency disease
- ocular conditions that may predispose the patient to future complications (e.g., ker-

atoconus, recurrent corneal erosion syndrome, or corneal dystrophy)

Relative Contraindications
• pregnancy or nursing
• use of isotretinoin (Accutane; Roche Pharmaceuticals, Nutley, NJ), amiodarone (Cordarone, Wyeth-Ayerst Laboratories, Madison, NJ), and/or sumatriptan (Imitrex; Glaxo Wellcome, Inc., Research Triangle Park, NC)

Methods
• Administer topical anesthesia alone, topical anesthesia with mild short-acting sedation, or topical anesthesia with intravenous conscious sedation and local anesthesia.
• Prepare and drape the patient in the usual fashion for anterior segment surgery.
• Use tetracaine drops as required.
• Use "verbal" anesthesia (constant reassurance to the patient throughout the procedure).
• Use an 11-mm OZ marker to mark the geometric center to the cornea to ensure accurate placement of the incision.
• Soak a Chayet sponge with tetracaine before making the incision or just prior to placement of the vacuum centering guide (VCG).
• With a previously inked incision marker, delineate the position of the radial incision, which should be no more than 1.8 mm long.

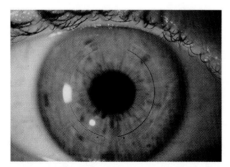

Figure 18–3 Appearance of Intacs after placement.

• Measure the peripheral corneal thickness at the center of the radial incision mark by ultrasound pachymetry, and set a diamond knife to 68% of this reading.
• Make a radial incision with the diamond knife at two-thirds of the corneal depth in the peripheral stroma.
• Using a modified Suarez spreader, laterally separate the corneal tissue at the base of the incision to prepare a corneal pocket near each side of the incision.
• Place a VCG over the center mark.
• Insert a dissector into the incision.
• Perform dissection of the cornea at two-thirds depth, clockwise and counterclockwise.
• Release the VCG.
• Use forceps to place the segments through the stromal channels.
• Position the segments temporally with a Sinskey (Duckworth's Kent, St. Louis, MO) hook so that the superior ends are approximately 3 mm apart and symmetrically positioned around the incisions.
• Appose the radial incision edges as indicated in Figure 18–3.
• Place sutures.
  ○ To close the incision, use one or two 11-0 nylon interrupted sutures (ensures good wound apposition through postoperative day 7).
  ○ Shorter incisions (<1.8 mm) may require placement of only one suture.
  ○ Remove sutures at postoperative day 7.
  ○ If you observe loose sutures or at least 1.0 D of suture-induced manifest refraction cylinder ("with the rule" astigmatism), remove sutures earlier.

Intraoperative Complications
• allergic reactions, the remote chance of damage to the eye, medical complications, or death from anesthesia
• see Table 18–1

TABLE 18–1
Intraoperative Complications

Possible Complications	Cause	Impact or Result	Prevention	Management
Marking the cornea				
Center mark improperly located	Did not locate geometric center	Decentered Intacs placement Intacs placement <1 mm from limbus	Use 11-mm zone marker	Re-mark geometric center
Center mark fades prior to application of VCG	Not enough pressure or ink	Unable to properly center VCG	Indent epithelium with Sinskey hook at geometric center. Apply ink to Sinskey hook	Re-mark geometric center
Smeared markings	Too much ink on I&P marker	Improper placement of incision or Intacs segments	Gentle application of ink to corneal marker	Maintain 1 mm between incision and limbus. Position superior segment ends ~3 mm apart and symmetrically around the incision
Diamond knife incision				
Shallow incision	Knife set incorrectly Inconsistent pressure during incision	Shallow pocketing and/or shallow dissection that could lead to corneal surface perforation	Consider use of Micron Scope to verify knife setting, which should be 68% of intraoperative pachymetry reading or ≥0.410 mm. Use "push-hold-cut" technique (apply firm, consistent pressure to footplate through entire incision; pause for 3-count after initial plunge)	Verify knife blade setting Recut incision
Deep incision	Knife set incorrectly	Anterior chamber perforation	Consider use of Micron Scope to verify knife setting	Stop the procedure immediately
Incision too long	Incision started or ended beyond incision mark	Incision <1 mm from limbus could lead to limbal bleeding and postoperative neovascularization. Enlarged postoperative epithelial defect	Trace entire length of incision mark only	Use NeoSynephrine 2.5% (Mydfrin; Alcon Laboratories, Fort Worth, TX) for limbal bleeding Avoid extra manipulation of incision edges

Incision too short	Incision started or ended prior to full length of incision mark	Glides do not fit, cannot initiate dissection	Trace entire length of incision mark	Enlarge incision to full length of incision mark
Pocketing technique				
Wound maceration	Stretching the wound or incision edges / Using instruments on the incision edges	Epithelial trauma / Postoperative induced astigmatism	Avoid excessive manipulation of incision edges including stretching and use of instruments, such as forceps, on the incision edges	Rehydrate incision / Inspect incision site carefully to assess damage / Consider not placing Intacs
Shallow pockets	Pocket initiated above base of incision	Excessive resistance to intrastromal tunnel dissection. Tissue wave in front of dissector. Shallow dissection leading to corneal surface perforation. Misaligned pockets leading to Intacs placement on different stromal levels	Initiate pockets at full depth of incision on both sides of incision and within a single intrastromal plane	Repocket at base of incision and within a single intrastromal plane
Deep pockets	Pocket initiated beneath base of incision	Anterior chamber perforation	*Do not* insert Sinskey hook or pocketing hook "tip down" into the incision / Always enter incision with blunt edges of instruments	Stop the procedure immediately
Narrow pockets	Pockets do not extend the full length of the incision	Glides do not fit in pockets	Initiate pockets to be as wide as the full incision length and to extend the full length of the stromal spreader blade	Repocket with stromal spreader
Application of VCG				
Chemosis	Draping technique / Use of local anesthesia / Use of pilocarpine / Prolonged manipulation or exposure to VCG	Loss of suction / Decentered or elongated tunnels	Avoid traumatic draping / Avoid use of anesthetic injections / Avoid use of pilocarpine / Limit continuous application of VCG to 3 min;before allow 5-min rest period reestablishing suction	"Milk" chemosis with VCG / Gently press VCG to globe while applying suction / If significant chemosis occurs, consider rescheduling surgery

Continued on next page

TABLE 18–1 (Continued)

Intraoperative Complications

Possible Complications	Cause	Impact or Result	Prevention	Management
Subconjunctival hemorrhage	Repeated application of VCG Manipulation of conjunctiva using forceps	Loss of suction	Limit continuous application of VCG to 3 min; allow 5-min rest period before reestablishing suction. Avoid manipulating conjunctiva with forceps or other instruments	Massage swollen conjunctival tissue with VCG Gently press VCG to globe while applying suction If significant, consider rescheduling surgery
Inadequate suction or break in suction leading to loss of centration	Improper placement of VCG Excessive downward pressure on dissector Pressure to side of globe	Elliptical intrastromal tunnel dissection leading to improper placement of Intacs and possibly poor visual outcomes for the patient	After ensuring proper centration, apply gentle downward pressure as suction is initiated Position VCG port temporarily to avoid suction break because of unexpected contact with tubing Do not press down or lift up on dissector during tunnel dissection	Always recenter using I&P Marker Allow 5-min rest period before reestablishing suction If unable to reestablish good suction, reschedule surgery
Intrastromal tunnel dissection				
Shallow dissection	Shallow pocket	Excessive resistance to intrastromal tunnel dissection. Tissue wave in front of dissector. Corneal surface perforation	Ensure appropriate pocket depth before beginning dissections	Stop dissection, repocket at base of incision and retunnel Assess corneal surface perforation and either repocket and retunnel or reschedule surgery
Deep dissection	Deep or perforated pocket	Anterior chamber perforation	Ensure appropriate pocket depth before beginning dissections	Stop surgery immediately if an anterior chamber perforation occurs
Misaligned, decentered or elliptical tunnels	Decentration of VCG Loss of suction	Poor visual outcomes for the patient from elliptical or decentered tunnels, inferior or superior displacement of tunnels, or nasal or temporal displacement of tunnels	Ensure proper centration of VCG before and after suction has been applied Do not push down or raise up on dissectors during dissection Position VCG port temporarily Do not continue dissection if suction is lost	Break suction and recenter VCG using corneal marker Attempt to retunnel Stop the procedure

Intacs placement

Introduction of bacteria to intrastromal tunnel	Contact by Intacs or surgical instruments with corneal surface or lid margins prior to placement	*Do not allow Intacs segments or surgical instruments to contact the corneal surface or lid margins prior to placement*	Infection	Manage infections
Positioning hole located inferiorly	Improper placement of segment	Ensure proper segment orientation prior to placement. Follow direction arrows on Intacs package	May make segment removal or repositioning more difficult	Remove segment and reposition
Elliptical placement of Intacs segments	Improper placement of segments	"Push out and twist" when placing Intacs segment to ensure segment is aligned with outer edge of placement marking	Poor visual outcomes for the patient	Remove segment and reposition
Intacs upside down	Improper alignment of segment cone angle	Verify segment position in forceps prior to placement	Difficult to insert segment	Remove segment, verify segment position in forceps, and reposition
Inadequate inferior dissection	Incomplete rotation of dissector	Rotate dissector full length of blade until support spoke contacts the incision edge	Proper positioning of segments cannot be achieved. Segments may migrate under incision	Reapply vacuum and retunnel to full length of dissector blade
Smeared or faded segment position markings	Too much or not enough ink on I&P marker	Gently apply ink to I&P marker	Proper position of segments difficult	Position superior segment ends ~3 mm apart and symmetrically around the incision
Incision closure				
Tight closure	Overtensioned suture(s)	Hydrate incision to approximate edges. Recommend using 11-0 interrupted suture. Make sure incision edges are apposed at the end of the procedure. Avoid overtensioning suture(s)	Suture-induced astigmatism	Remove suture if postoperative astigmatism is observed
Loose closure	Loose or missing suture(s). Incision edges not properly approximated	Hydrate incision to approximate edges. Suture if necessary	Incision gape. Epithelial cysts or plugs	Place one or two interrupted 11-0 nylon suture(s)

POSTOPERATIVE CONSIDERATIONS

Postoperative visits are usually scheduled for 1 day, 1 week, 1 month, 3 months, and 6 months after surgery.

Day of Surgery
- expected symptoms
  - mild to moderate discomfort/pain for a few hours after surgery (if pain is more severe, contact the surgeon)
  - foreign body sensation or "scratchiness" (common during the immediate postoperative period)
  - fluctuating vision during the first month
  - dry eyes for the first 2 to 3 months
- management
  - Apply an antibiotic-steroid combination ointment or solution (0.1% dexamethasone and 0.3% tobramycin or equivalent) to the operative eye at the end of the procedure.
  - Perform a slit-lamp examination (to observe the segment placement and incision closure and to verify tunnel depth).
  - Cover the operative eye with a clear shield (the patient should wear a shield at night for 1 week).
  - Provide the patient with postoperative instructions.
  - Prescribe analgesic medication (acetaminophen, paracetamol, or equivalent) for postoperative discomfort (prescribe other pain medication at your discretion).
  - Provide artificial tears as needed.
  - Recommend that the patient take a nap (patients will be photophobic and they should rest their eyes).
  - Prescribe postoperative medications [antibiotic-steroid combination solution (0.1% dexamethasone/0.3% tobramycin or equivalent], four times a day for 1 week.
  - Instruct the patient to watch for symptoms of infection (e.g., dull, aching pain or discomfort, with or without photophobia) at any point in the postoperative period.
  - Remind the patient to contact his or her doctor if any of these symptoms occur.
  - Advise the patient to avoid rubbing the eye (may lead to segment migration or improper healing of the incision).

The Immediate Postoperative Period (Days 1–7)
Expected Results
- good visual acuity (majority of patients see better than 20/40)
  - Advise patient that over the next 3 to 6 weeks visual acuity will be good but may fluctuate from day to day and even during the course of the day.
  - Advise patient who does not have 20/40 vision that refractive surgery procedures typically require some recovery time and that vision will most likely improve.
- good intraocular pressure
- possible astigmatism
  - No intervention is necessary.
- epithelium healing
  - Healing is usually complete and foreign-body sensation resolved by the end of the first week.

COMPLICATIONS Several complications may be observed during the first week of postoperative recovery.

Epithelial Defect
- usually measures about 2 × 2 mm at the end of surgery
- rare incidence of adverse events (1.1% during U.S. clinical trials)
- symptoms
  - decreased visual acuity (usually slightly less at day 3 than on day 1, secondary to superficial punctate keratitis from the

topical medications and increased suture-induced astigmatism as the superior corneal edema in the region of the incision resolves)
  ○ diurnal fluctuating vision (usually reported by patient because he or she generally self-tests his own visual acuity in the operative eye 6–20 times per day)
  ○ pain (but no patient discomfort from a peri-incisional epithelial defect located under the upper lid)
  ○ foreign body sensation (if epithelium has not yet healed)
  ○ photophobia
• findings
  ○ possible mild subconjunctival hemorrhage and/or chemosis remaining from the VCG
  ○ little to no intraocular inflammation
• management
  ○ Half of cases almost entirely resolve by the first postoperative day and most others completely resolve by day 3.
  ○ Attempt to bury suture knots, if not already done.
  ○ Provide a bandage contact lens to be worn until the defect heals.
  ○ If the epithelial defect is larger than 2 × 2 mm, use a bandage contact lens or mild patching. (Beware of excessive pressure on the dome of the cornea that could cause movement or malpositioning of the segments.)
  ○ Monitor bandage contact lens use (prolonged contact lens wear may aggravate superficial neovascularization to the superior aspect of the incision).
  ○ Discontinue the bandage contact lens as soon as the epithelial defect resolves or when limbal vascular buds form.

Filamentary Keratitis
• usually a single filament extending from the end of the incision (causes disproportionate discomfort to the patient)

• symptoms
  ○ foreign body sensation
  ○ photophobia
• findings
  ○ occasionally may develop as the epithelial defect heals
• management
  ○ Treat with debridement, hypertonic saline drops (5% sodium chloride), or a bandage contact lens.
  ○ See Epithelial Defects section for information about monitoring and removing bandage contact lenses.

Drug Toxicity and Allergies
• symptoms
  ○ foreign body sensation
  ○ eye irritation
• findings
  ○ superficial punctate keratitis
  ○ extensive chemosis [possible allergic reaction to topical medications unless surgery involved significant trauma (i.e., difficulty with VCG placement or prolonged application of the VCG)]
  ○ lid edema
  ○ lid erythema
• management
  ○ In the presence of severe conjunctival chemosis in the early postoperative period, shift topical medications to an increased dose of topical steroids.

Infection
• symptoms
  ○ significant ocular discomfort or pain
  ○ photophobia
  ○ decreased vision
  ○ ocular discomfort and photophobia (one patient in U.S. clinical trials for PMA Cohort who had infectious lamellar infiltrates)
• findings
  ○ infiltrate at incision
  ○ infiltrate in tunnel

◦ cultured *Staphyloccus epidermidis* (in the one case where an infectious infiltrate was identified in the U.S. clinical trials for the PMA Cohort, which suggests that it may have been introduced at the time of surgery, perhaps because of contact of the Intacs or instruments with the lid margin or the "lacrimal lake")
- management
  ◦ See all patients who call with complaints of rapid onset of discomfort and photophobia as soon as possible.
  ◦ Suspect infection in rapidly progressive infiltrates that appear in the first or second postoperative week.
  ◦ Manage infiltrates that progress more rapidly, however, with aggressive topical fortified broad-spectrum antibiotic therapy.
  ◦ If the infiltrates progress more slowly, fortified topical antibiotic therapy and systemic antibiotic therapy may lead to quick resolution.
  ◦ Consider removal of Intacs.

Corneal Edema
- peripheral or central corneal edema and recurrent or extended corneal edema (rare)
- mild corneal edema from placement, removal, or replacement of Intacs or other refractive procedures (routine)
- symptoms
  ◦ blurred vision
- management
  ◦ Prescribe or increase the dosage of topical corticosteroids.

Suture-Induced Astigmatism
- symptoms (associated with induced astigmatism or undercorrection)
  ◦ glare
  ◦ halos
  ◦ double images
  ◦ blurred vision

- findings
  ◦ with the rule astigmatism (not coupled)
  ◦ steepening along the 90-degree meridian, which leads to additional steepening along the 180-degree meridian (perhaps from blunting of the typical flattening that occurs in the opposite meridian with suture-induced astigmatism)
  ◦ For example, a $-2.00 + 2.00 \times 90$-degree refraction prior to suture removal shifts to plano after suture removal.
  ◦ undercorrection
  ◦ use of 10-0 nylon, more than one suture, tight suture closure, wound dehydration during surgery, and wound maceration or excess manipulation during surgery (all increase risk)
- management
  ◦ If induced astigmatism is at least 1.00 D, identify the probable source of the astigmatism.
  ◦ Astigmatism related to over-tensioning of the incision sutures (i.e., with the rule astigmatism) typically diminishes over time.
  ◦ If there is more than 1.00 D with the rule astigmatism and sutures are still in place after day 7, remove the sutures.
  ◦ Address suture-induced astigmatism early if the incision is healed and does not stain with fluorescein.

The Intermediate Postoperative Period (Weeks 1–4)
Expected Results
- no ocular discomfort or inflammation
- uncorrected visual acuity (UCVA) typically better than 20/40 (fluctuates from day to day and during the course of a day, usually in proportion with the induced astigmatism)

COMPLICATIONS Several complications do not become apparent until later during recovery.

Induced With-the-Rule Astigmatism

- a myopic shift in the spherical equivalent (Intacs may blunt the concomitant flattening usually seen with suture-induced astigmatism)
- symptoms
  - astigmatic blur
  - double vision
- findings
  - a long incision with limbal encroachment
  - visible incision and suture scarring
  - elliptical decentration
  - with the rule topographic changes
  - too tight sutures or those left in place too long (according to current clinical data, may result in prolonged or even permanent with-the-rule astigmatism, even after suture removal)
- management
  - Administer topical corticosteroids to carefully modulate overly aggressive wound healing during the initial postoperative period.
  - Reincise the original incision and suture loosely or leave the incision unsutured for those patients who have corneas that healed aggressively. (This strategy has had only very limited success in a very small number of patients with astigmatism. Available clinical data have not demonstrated consistent results.)
  - Selective suture removal may be necessary if the induced astigmatism is greater than 1.00 D at 2 weeks.
  - Remove sutures by 4 weeks.

Induced "Against-the-Rule" Astigmatism

- symptoms
  - double vision
  - astigmatic blur
- findings
  - "against-the-rule" topographic changes
  - incision wound gape
  - cysts

- epithelial plugs
- inadequate wound closure
- wound trauma (e.g., blunt force or eye rubbing)
- flatter than average preoperative asphericity
- management
  - Remove any epithelial cysts or plugs.
  - Debride the incision or reapproximate the wound edges and resuture the wound as appropriate.

Corneal Thinning

- symptoms
  - foreign body sensation
- findings
  - epithelial breakdown or staining over Intacs
  - shallow Intacs placement (typically when placed at <30% depth)
- management
  - Recommend early intervention to prevent corneal thinning.
  - Remove Intacs immediately.
- Make a new intrastromal tunnel at the appropriate depth (68% of pachymetry reading).
- Reposition Intacs.

Infiltrates

- may be infectious or sterile
  - see Infection on pp. 207–208
  - sterile infiltrates usually observed between day 14 and week 6
- symptoms
  - eye redness
  - photophobia
- findings
  - focal whitish infiltrate
  - iritis
  - epithelial streaming
  - poor wound healing
  - incomplete wound closure
  - presence of a foreign body (e.g., stromal debris, fiber)

○ inadequate steroid dosing

○ mechanical trauma

• management

○ Administer combined antibiotic and steroid treatment (even though some may self-resolve over time).

Intacs Displacement

• may be vertical or lateral

• symptoms

○ glare

○ starbursting

○ halo

○ variable visual acuity

• findings

○ inferior or superior placement or irregular astigmatism (vertical displacement)

○ inadequate centration mark during surgery, incomplete tunnel dissection, incomplete advancement of Intacs, aggressive eye rubbing by patient, or segment movement within the intrastromal tunnel (vertical decentration)

○ mismatched pupil center to surgical center of the Intacs, irregular topography, or irregular astigmatism (lateral displacement)

○ decentered intrastromal tunnel, poor VCG placement or loss of suction during surgery, aggressive eye rubbing by patient, oversized pocket superiorly, or removal of Intacs and replacement with segment movement within the intrastromal tunnel (lateral decentration)

• management

○ Replace Intacs and properly align the new lens on the pupillary center.

Large Pupils

• symptoms

○ Intacs edge visible to patient

○ glare

○ starbursting

• findings

○ large pupil in dark environment

○ mismatched pupil to surgical center of Intacs

○ poor Intacs placement

○ decentered intrastromal tunnel

○ segment movement within the intrastromal tunnel

• management

○ Carefully select patients to avoid large-pupil issues.

○ Remove or reposition the Intacs if decentration is the main issue (may self-resolve over time).

Epithelial Plug Formation in Incision

• management

○ Intervene as soon as possible after observing the plug.

○ Remove the incision sutures (if present) and debride and resuture the incision area.

○ Follow the patient closely for 2 weeks to ensure adequate incision closure.

The Late Postoperative Period (Month 2 and Beyond)

Between months 1 and 3 the surgeon should begin assessing whether the patient is satisfied with his or her vision and is "20/Happy." Follow satisfied patients on a routine basis after the six-month examination.

Expected Results

• stabilized visual acuity by month 3

• refractive stability typically maintained after month 3 (usually <1.00 D of shift in the spherical equivalent between subsequent visits)

• gradual resolution of any induced astigmatism (high degrees of cylinder should continue to resolve over time)

• positioning hole deposits (nonprogressive and clinically inconsequential)

○ usually appear 3 to 6 weeks postoperatively

○ filling of a small manipulation hole used for final positioning of Intacs at the superior end of each Intacs segment with an opalescent substance (documented on a limited basis as proteoglycan, collagen, and keratocytes)

COMPLICATIONS In general, late complications of Intacs placement are rare.

Intrastromal Tunnel Deposits
- generally appear between 3 and 12 months postoperatively
- findings
  - observed in 68% of the U.S. Phase III clinical trial patients at the month 12 exam
  - remain confined to the intrastromal tunnel (do not spread centrally into the visual axis)
  - rarely, lead to confluent accumulations of opalescent material limited entirely to the dissected intrastromal tunnel
  - may become visible to the naked eye
  - from month 6 to month 12, prevalence and levels of deposits remain stable
  - causes not yet conclusively established

Pannus and Deep Neovascularization
- findings
  - prior contact lens wear
  - preoperative pannus
  - incision extending to the limbal vessels during surgery
  - wound healing issues (e.g., neovascularization in incision)
  - loose sutures

Undercorrection or Overcorrection
- findings
  - vessel growth
- management
  - Before considering replacement, perform a cycloplegic refraction and evaluate topography.
  - Where appropriate, discuss options including replacement.

- Prescribe topical corticosteroids to stop vessel growth once present.
- Advanced vessel growth that does not respond to topical corticosteroids may require laser therapy to impede deep vessel growth.
- Replace Intacs with thinner or thicker segments, depending on the residual refractive error (currently, insufficient data on efficacy of exchanging Intacs)
- Remove Intacs.
- See section on Removal and Replacement that follows.

Removal and Replacement
Intacs may be removed or replaced, unlike essentially permanent refractive techniques that directly cut or remove tissue and may be adjusted but not undone. Initial results of Intacs removal are very good although further analysis is needed. In FDA trials, only 6.9% of patients required removal in the first year.

Indications
- change in patient's vision over time
- a clinically significant complication
- titration of the refractive effect with thicker or thinner Intacs

Expected Results
- within one line of preoperative BCVA
- no complications
- return of refraction to preoperative levels within 3 months (most cases)
- an additional effect because of replacement with thicker segments (6 procedures in FDA study)

Methods
- Set an adjustable-depth diamond knife to a setting that corresponds to the Intacs depth that was estimated during slit-lamp examination and/or optical pachymetry.

- Make a single cut-down incision, approximately 1.8 mm in length (the incision may be at or very near the original entry incision), through the epithelium and stroma down to the level of Intacs.
- Place the incision approximately 1 mm away from any vascularization in the limbal region.
- Use D&K titanium Sinskey hooks because of their stiffness (stainless-steel Sinskey hooks are not as effective).
- For Intacs that have been in place for a short time, reopen the original entry incision to full depth with a Sinskey hook or similar instrument.
- Using a stromal spreader, Sinskey hook, or similar instrument, repocket to expose the original channel to the proximal end of the Intacs.
- Clear a path around the entire end of the segment with a Sinskey hook.
- Break free any fibrous ingrowth that may have occurred by running the Sinskey hook over and under the positioning hole of the Intacs, being careful not to snag the stroma.
- "Wiggle" the segment while attempting to pull continuously in a tangential direction to the circumference of the segment.
- difficult cases
  - Gently massage the surface of the cornea to manipulate the segment and loosen adhesion within the channel.
  - Apply constant moderate force and wiggle the hook to manipulate the segment and loosen adhesion within the channel.
  - Probe the channel with a blunt instrument or Sinskey hook, along the outside edge of the segment, to break stroma free from the Intacs surface.
  - As a last resort, consider placing new incisions near the proximal end of the Intacs segment or an inferior incision to gain access to the distal segment end to facilitate removal.

- Placement of new incisions near the 1:00 and 11:00 positions prohibits an Intacs exchange procedure because Intacs segment ends lie near the new incisions.
- Rotate Intacs within the tunnel to expose the end of the segment at the incision.
- Grasp the segment with Intacs forceps and remove by rotating out through the reopened entry incision.

ALTERNATIVE TREATMENTS

Intacs insertion is the first new refractive surgery technology to appear since laser in situ keratomileusis (LASIK), photorefractive keratectomy (PRK), and radial keratotomy (RK). LASIK, PRK, and RK were originally used to treat higher myopic patients, leaving patients with low myopia with very low hopes for laser vision correction.

The use of Intacs, LASIK, and intraocular lenses (IOLs) will most likely overlap somewhat, just as glasses, contact lenses, and refractive surgery have. Surgeons may choose among them based on their skill level, patient profiles, and practice environment.

Laser In Situ Keratomileusis

There has been no formal study of LASIK after initial Intacs insertion or LASIK and then subsequent insertion of Intacs, and no supporting data are available. However, anecdotal reports suggest that LASIK is effective after Intacs removal.

Characteristics
- similarities with Intacs
  - use of topical anesthesia
  - comparable visual results

- dissimilarities with Intacs
  - ability of Intacs to be placed (and if necessary, removed or replaced) without disturbing the visual axis
  - better quality of vision with Intacs according to available single-site data

Suggested Readings

Asbell PA, Ucakhan OO, Durrie DS, Lindstrom RL. Adjustability of refractive effect for corneal ring segments. *J Refract Surg.* 1999;15:627–631.

Burris TE, Baker PC, Ayer CT, et al. Flattening of central corneal curvature with intrastromal corneal rings of increasing thickness: an eye-bank eye study. *Cataract Refract Surg.* 1993;9(suppl):182–187.

Fleming JF, Lovisolo CF. Intrastromal corneal ring segments in a patient with previous laser in situ keratomileusis. *J Refract Surg.* 2000;16: 365–367.

Twa MD, Hurst TJ, Walker JG, Waring GO, Schanzlin DJ. Diurnal stability of refraction after implantation with intracorneal ring segments. *J Cataract Refract Surg.* 2000;26:516–523.

Twa MD, Karpecki PM, King BJ, Linn SH, Durrie DS, Schanzlin DJ. One-year results from the phase III investigation of the KeraVision Intacs. *J Am Optom Assoc.* 1999;70:515–524.

CHAPTER 19

Surgical Reversal of Presbyopia

John F. Doane

CHAPTER CONTENTS

Ideally, visual function after age 40 would allow individuals to have excellent unaided distance and near vision with identical distance and near focal points in each eye. This level of visual function is what non-presbyopic emmetropic patients enjoy—unifocal vision (symmetrical focal points for each eye) with variable focality (the ability to focus distant, intermediate, and near targets). Presbyopic individuals do not have this level of visual function.

If any refractive error has defied surgical correction to date, it is presbyopia. Options for management include
- spectacles (bifocal, trifocal, progressive, and reader)
- contact lenses (monovision, bifocal, and multifocal)
- intraocular lenses (IOLs) (monovision, multifocal, and accommodating)
- corneal refractive surgery (monovision or multifocal ablations)

In general, none of these options are universally accepted by all patients. A majority of the population may tolerate each technique, but significant proportions of the population do not fully accept them.

MONOVISION

The most commonly performed technique for managing presbyopia has been the induction of monovision (the intentional targeting of a small amount of myopia in one eye to facilitate near and intermediate visual tasks).

Advantages
- patient satisfaction of about 50% (tolerance by 25–30% and the remainder abhorrence)

Disadvantages
- spatial "dizziness"
- nausea
- distance blurring
- night time glare, halos, or starbursting
- depth perception difficulties

MULTIFOCAL APPROACHES

- multifocal contact lenses
- bifocal contact lenses
- multifocal ablations

Advantages
- greater range of useable visual acuity over far, intermediate, and near distances than monofocal corrections

Disadvantages
- ghost images
- glare
- haloing
- worsening of visual disturbances in low-light situations
- an unacceptable trade-off between greater range of focus and slightly reduced best acuity at a distance and near compared with monofocal options (for some patients)

ACCOMMODATING TECHNIQUES

Accommodating techniques such as pseudophakic accommodating IOLs are currently being investigated. The work is in the very early stages, but this type of correction would allow for a unifocal lens with variable focality.

SURGICAL REVERSAL OF PRESBYOPIA

Ronald Schachar, M.D., developed a technique for the surgical reversal of presbyopia (SRP) using scleral expansion band segments.

In theory, this method facilitates accommodation without compromising distance uncorrected visual acuity (UCVA). Schachar's surgical procedure is designed to

expand the diameter of the eye overlying the ciliary muscle.

Theories of Accommodation with Presbyopia

Schachar's model for the loss of accommodation with age diametrically opposes Helmholz's theory. However, recent experimental evidence that supports Helmholtz's original theory challenges Schachar's theory.

Helmholz's Theory
- The crystalline lens loses its flexibility.
- The lens does not increase its converging power with relaxation of the ciliary muscle to facilitate near-vision tasks as it did before age 40.

Schachar's Theory
- Presbyopia with age results from physiologic growth of the crystalline lens of the eye (Fig. 19–1).
- The increase in the size of the crystalline lens reduces the distance between the edge of the crystalline lens and the ciliary muscle.
- The ciliary muscle, which changes the shape of the crystalline lens by traction on the zonules, is unable to exert sufficient force to alter the shape of the lens.

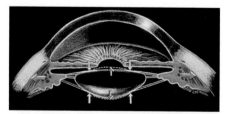

Figure 19–1 Animated view of Schachar's accommodative theory. With increasing radial tension on the zonules, the anterior and posterior crystalline lens radii of curvatures are decreased, which effectively increases the converging power of the crystalline lens. Thus, the lens accommodates for near-vision tasks.

- When this area expands it increases the distance between the ciliary muscle and the edge of the crystalline lens, permitting the ciliary muscle to exert more force on the lens, thus reestablishing accommodation.

Preoperative Considerations

Indications and Inclusion Criteria
- presbyopia
- healthy conjunctiva and sclera
- near emmetropic refractive error

Exclusion Criteria
- thin sclera
- cataract (cataract surgery should be performed when appropriate instead of scleral segment implants)
- a glaucoma-filtering bleb

Patient Evaluation
- Complete the standard refractive surgery evaluation per Chapters 4 to 7.
- We anticipate that the candidate is emmetropic for distance correction.
- Perform slit-lamp evaluation.
- Ensure that no scleral thinning is present.

Surgical Considerations

Methods
- Perform the surgery in an outpatient setting.
- Administer an oral systemic sedative (Valium or Versed).

- Mark the limbus at the 12:00 position.
- Prepare the skin with betadine.
- Administer topical proparacaine 0.5%.
- Drape the patient.
- Insert the speculum.
- Mark the cornea at 45-degree meridians.
- Make 5-mm arcuate conjunctival incisions 5.0 to 5.5 mm posterior to the limbus and centered at the 45-degree meridians.
- Dissect down to the bare sclera.
- Make two 900-μm-long, 300-μm-deep partial thickness incisions radially in each 45-degree meridian with the PRESBY (Presby Corpration) square guarded incisional diamond knife.
- Make the two incisions parallel to each other and separated by 4.5 mm.
- Straddle the incisions over the selected 45-degree meridian.
- Use a PRESBY lamellar diamond knife to create a scleral "belt loop" (900 μm wide and 300 μm deep) between the two radial incisions.
- Insert the PRESBY scleral segments in each quadrant (Figs. 19–2 and 19–3).
- Close the conjunctival incisions with 10-0 suture.

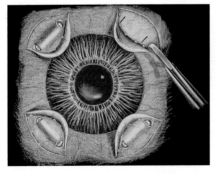

Figure 19–2 Insertion of band segment into "belt loop."

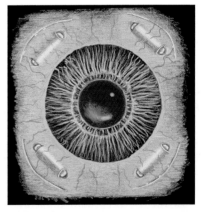

Figure 19–3 Four band segments are placed in each oblique quadrant and the overlying conjunctiva has been repositioned.

- Place one drop of pilocarpine 2% and two drops of a combination antibiotic steroid (e.g., Tobradex; Alcon, Forth Worth, TX) on the cornea.
- Administer 500 cc of intravenous mannitol (Osmitrol or Mannitol; Abbott Laboratories, Abbott Park, IL) within 30 min to shrink the vitreous volume and prevent marked rise in intraocular pressure after surgery.

Postoperative Considerations
Complications
- infection
- implant extrusion
- persistent conjunctival defect over implant
- scleral erosion
- anterior segment ischemia

Patient Care and Follow-Up
- Instruct the patient to use a topical antibiotic-steroid for 7 days and artificial tears and a lubricating ointment before sleep for at least 3 weeks.
- Remove nonabsorbable sutures that were used to close the conjunctiva 7 days postoperatively.
- Advise the patient to avoid eye rubbing.
- Instruct the patient to do pencil pushup and accommodative exercises daily.

Suggested Readings

Glasser A. Can accommodation be surgically restored in human presbyopia? *Optom Vis Sci.* 1999;76:607–608.

Glasser A, Kaufman PL. The mechanism of accommodation in primates. *Ophthalmology.* 1999;106:863–872.

Schachar RA, Cudmore DP, Black TD. Experimental support for Schachar's hypothesis of accommodation. *Ann Ophthalmol.* 1993;25: 404–409.

Schachar RA, Tello C, Cudmore DP, Liebmann JM, Black TD, Ritch R. In vivo increase of the human lens equatorial diameter during accommodation. *Am J Physiol.* 1996; 271:R670–R676.

INDEX

B-scan ultrasonography, indications and techniques, 62
Buratto technique, laser in situ keratomileusis (LASIK), 114–117

C

Cataract surgery
  vs. implantable contact lens (ICL) surgery, 175
  laser in situ keratomileusis following, 141
Central islands, formation of, with LASIK, 133–134
Centrifugal incision, radial keratotomy (RK) and, 74–75
Chalazion, refractive surgery contraindicated with, 23
Charge coupled device (CCD), Shack-Hartmann wavefront analysis system, 147
Chayet's astigmatism nomogram, photorefractive keratectomy (PRK), 85
Chromatic ocular aberrations, characteristics of, 144
Clear lens replacement
  advantages and disadvantages, 4, 153–154
  as alternative to photorefractive keratectomy (PRK), 86
  laser in situ keratomileusis (LASIK) and, 141, 158–159
  lens selection, 155–156
  postoperative management, 157–159
  preoperative assessment, 154–156
  surgical technique, 156–157
Coaxial light source incision, refractive surgery, 71
Collagen vascular disease
  preoperative assessment of, 33
  refractive surgery in patients with, 12
Colvard pupillometer, 42
Coma, optical aberrations, 145
Combined (genesis) technique, radial keratotomy (RK), 74–75
Complications
  clear lens replacement refractive surgery, 157–158
  Intacs corneal ring segment
    corneal edema, 207
    corneal thinning, 209
    displacement, 210
    drug toxicity and allergies, 207
    epithelial defect, 206–207
    epithelial plug formation, 210
    filamentary keratitis, 207
    induced against-the-rule astigmatism, 209
    induced with-the-rule astigmatism, 208
    infection, 207–208
    infiltrates, 209–210
    intraoperative, 201–205
    intrastromal tunnel deposits, 211

large pupils, 210
    pannus and deep neovascularization, 211
    postoperative, 206–211
    suture-induced astigmatism, 207
    under- or over-correction, 211
  iris-claw phakic intraocular lens insertion (IOL)
    perioperative complications, 170–172
    postoperative complications, 172–173
  laser in situ keratomileusis (LASIK)
    astigmatism irregularities, 134–136
    central island formations, 133–134
    corneal neovascularization, 122–123
    corneal perforation, 123–124
    decentered ablations, 136–137
    dislodged flap, 128–129
    epithelial defects, 124–126
    epithelial ingrowth, 129–130
    flap complications, 121–122
    infection, 127–128
    interface debris, 129
    LASIK interface keratitis (LIK), 125–127
    postoperative pain, 124
    refractive outcome errors, 131–132
  limbal relaxing incisions (LRI), 79–80
  noncontact laser thermal keratoplasty studies, 98–99
  phakic intraocular lens insertion (IOL), 164–165
  phakic refractive lens implantation, 192–193
  photorefractive keratectomy (PRK) postoperative management, 87–88
  posterior-chamber implantable contact lens, 180, 182–183
  radial keratotomy (RK), 76–77
  surgical reversal of presbyopia, 217
Compound astigmatism, photorefractive keratectomy (PRK), 85
Computerized corneal topography, postoperative assessment with, 55–58
Computerized videokeratography (CVK), noncontact laser thermal keratoplasty studies, 96–98
Conjunctival abnormalities, refractive surgery for, 23–24
Conjunctival chemosis, characteristics of, 23
Contact laser thermal keratoplasty (LTK), indications and techniques for, 93–94
Contact lenses, risks and problems with, 29–30
Contrast sensitivity testing, indications and techniques for, 63
Corneal disorders
  refractive surgery for, 15–21
    endothelial disorders, 21
    epithelial disorders, 15–17
    stromal disorders, 17–21
  slit-lamp examination of, 42–43

Corneal edema, as Intacs corneal ring segment complication, 208

Corneal neovascularization
as Intacs corneal ring segment complication, 211
laser in situ keratomileusis (LASIK), 122–123
refractive surgery for patients with, 16–17

Corneal perforation, laser in situ keratomileusis (LASIK), 123–124

Corneal thickness measurements, refractive surgery and, 19

Corneal thinning, as Intacs corneal ring segment complication, 209

Corrective lenses, preoperative assessment of prior refractive history, 33

Corticosteroids, photorefractive keratectomy (PRK) postoperative management, 86–87

Cosmetic and personal needs, refractive surgery preoperative assessment, 29–30

Cost issues, with refractive surgery, 31

Crossed-cylinder ablation, laser in situ keratomileusis (LASIK), 119–120

Cryolathe techniques, freeze keratomileusis and, 103–104

Cycloplegic retinoscopy, refractive error measurements, 53–54

Curvature of field, characteristics of, 145

Custom cornea measurement device, components of, 150–151

D

Decentered ablations, as LASIK complication, 136–137

Diabetes mellitus, refractive surgery in patients with, 11–12

Diamond knife, incisional refractive techniques using, 70–72, 74

Distometer, trial frame refraction measurements, 52

Distortion, optical aberrations and, 145

Doane-Slade superior hinge technique, laser in situ keratomileusis (LASIK), 119–120

Dresden wavefront analyzer, components of, 151

Drug toxicity, as Intacs corneal ring segment complication, 207

E

Electro-optical ray-tracing analyzer, components of, 152

Emmetropia, classification and characteristics, 5–6

Endocrine disorders, refractive surgery in patients with, 14–15

Endothelial guttata, 21, 43

Environmental factors, refractive disorder epidemiology and, 9

Epikeratophakia, techniques and indications for, 108–109

Epithelial basement membrane dystrophy (EBMD), refractive surgery for patients with, 15–16

Epithelial defects
epithelial ingrowth, 129–131
ingrowth, LASIK complications with, 129–131
as Intacs corneal ring segment complication, 206–207
laser in situ keratomileusis (LASIK), 124–126
refractive surgery for patients with, 15–17

Epithelial plug, as Intacs corneal ring segment complication, 210

Ethnicity, myopia prevalence and, 9

Extraocular muscles, refractive surgery for, 24–25

Eye dominance testing, 37–38

Eyelid abnormalities, 22–23, 26

Eye tracking, custom laser in situ keratomileusis (LASIK) with wavefront technology, 152

F

Family, preoperative assessment of, 32

Filimentary keratitis, as Intacs corneal ring segment complication, 207

Financing options, for refractive surgery costs, 31

Fissure size, refractive surgery and, 26

Flap complications
dislodged flap, LASIK complication with, 128–129
laser in situ keratomileusis (LASIK), 121–122
LASIK flap striae, 127–128

Flap repositioning technique, laser in situ keratomileusis (LASIK), 119–120

Fleischer's ring, slit-lamp examination of, 43

Fogged alternate cover balance, refractive error measurement, 50–51

Fogged prism disassociated balance, refractive error measurement, 49

Foldable lenses, clear lens replacement refractive surgery, 155

Forme fruste keratoconus, computerized corneal topographic assessment of, 55

Four base out test, eye dominance, 38–39

Framing technique, eye dominance testing, 37–38

Freeze keratomileusis, disadvantages of, 102–104

Fuch's dystrophy, refractive surgery in patients with, 21

Fundus, examination of, 43–44

G

Gender, refractive disorder epidemiology, 9

Genetics, refractive disorder epidemiology, 9

Glaucoma, fundus examination with, 44

H

Halos, as photorefractive keratectomy (PRK) complication, 87, 89

Haptics, phakic intraocular lens insertion (IOL), 162–163

Hatsis classification, laser interface keratitis (LIK), 126

Haze, as photorefractive keratectomy (PRK) complication, 87–88

Helium-neon lasers, noncontact laser thermal keratoplasty, 95–98

Helmholz's theory, surgical reversal of presbyopia, 215

Herpes simplex, refractive surgery in patients with, 13

Herpes zoster, refractive surgery in patients with, 13

Herpetic keratitis, refractive surgery in patients with, 13

Higher-order optical aberrations, characteristics of, 145

High-frequency anterior segment ultrasound biomicroscopy, indications and techniques for, 62–63

Hole card, eye dominance testing, 37–38

Holium laser keratoplasty, as alternative to photorefractive keratectomy (PRK), 86

Holladay-Godwin pupil gauge, pupil assessment using, 42

Holladay refraction formula, phakic refractive lens implantation technique, 188

Holmium:yttrium-aluminum-garnet laser
  contact laser thermal keratoplasty, 93–94
  future applications and studies, 99
  noncontact laser thermal keratoplasty, 94–98
  techniques and applications, 92–93

Human immunodeficiency virus (HIV), refractive surgery in patients with, 12–13

Humphrey autorefractor, refrative error measurement, 45

Hyperopia
  binocular fog manifest refraction, 47
  classification and characteristics, 7
  iris-claw phakic intraocular lens insertion (IOL) for, 172
  laser in situ keratomileusis (LASIK), 115–116
  level of correction with refractive surgery, 31
  phakic refractive lens implantation, pediatric applications, 195–196
  photorefractive keratectomy (PRK), 84–85
  posterior-chamber implantable contact lens, 181–182

Hyperopic astigmatism, classification and characteristics, 7

Hyperopic automated lamellar keratoplasty, advantages and disadvantages, 3

Hypertension, refractive surgery in patients with, 10–11

I

Immersion A-scans, indications for, 61

Incisional refractive techniques, 68–80
  astigmatic keratotomy (AK), 77–78
  equipment for, 70
  limbal relaxing incisions (LRI), 79–80
  postoperative considerations, 72–73
  preoperative considerations, 68–69
  radial keratotomy (RK), 73–77
  surgical considerations, 69–72

Infection (postoperative), 127, 207–208

Infectious diseases, refractive surgery in patients with, 12–14, 33

Infiltrates, as Intacs corneal ring segment complication, 209–210

Inflammatory disorders, preoperative assessment of, 33

Informed consent, procedures in refractive surgery, 33–35

Intacs corneal ring segment, 198–213
  advantages, 199–200
  alternative treatments, 212–213
  complications
    intraoperative, 201–205
    postoperative, 206–211
  contraindications, 200–201
  history and evolution, 198–200
  indications and inclusion criteria for, 200
  patient education, 200
  patient preparation, 200
  postoperative management, 206–212
  preoperative assessment, 200
  removal and replacement, 211–212
  specifications, 199
  surgical considerations, 200–205

Interface debris, LASIK complications with, 129

Intracorneal ring (ICR). *See also* Intacs corneal ring segment as refractive surgery option, 1–2

Intraocular contact lens (ICL). *See also* Phakic intraocular lens; Posterior-chamber implantable contact lens
  high-frequency anterior segment ultrasound biomicroscopy and, 62
  phakic refractive lens implantation, piggybacking with, 196

Intraocular pressure (IOP), posterior-chamber implantable contact lens, postoperative treatment of, 180–181

Intrastromal tunnel deposits, as INTACS corneal ring segment complication, 211

IOL. *See* Intraocular contact lens (IOL)

PTK. *See* Phototherapeutic keratectomy (PTK)
Ptosis, refractive surgery for, 22
Pupil card, pupil size evaluation, 41
Pupillometry, preoperative assessment, 41–42
Pupil size
    enlargement, as Intacs corneal ring segment
        complication, 210
    optical aberrations and, 145
    pupillometric evaluation, 41–42
    refractive surgery and, 25

R
Radial astigmatism, characteristics of, 145
Radial keratotomy (RK)
    advantages and disadvantages, 1, 3
    complications, 75–76
    incisional refractive techniques, 73–77
        preoperative considerations, 73
        surgical considerations, 73–74
    laser in situ keratomileusis following, 137–139
    phototherapeutic keratectomy (PTK) after, 90–91
    postoperative considerations, 76–77
Recreational needs and restrictions, refractive
        surgery preoperative assessment, 29–30
Recurrent corneal erosion (RCE), refractive
        surgery in patients with, 16
Red-green prism disassociated duochrome bal-
        ance, refractive error measurement, 49–50
Refraction targets
    age concerns, 64–65
    bilateral distance target, 65–66
    bilateral near or intermediate target, 66
    monovision, 66–67
    multifocal lenses, 67
    surgical categories and techniques, 64
Refractive disorders
    classification and characteristics, 5–9
    pathologic ocular changes, 9
Refractive error
    evaluation of, 45–83
        astigmatism, 47–48
        binocular balancing, 48–50
        binocular fog manifest refraction, 46–47
        computerized corneal topography, 55–58
        contrast sensitivity testing, 63
        cycloplegic retinoscopy, 53–54
        high-frequency anterior segment ultrasound
            biomicroscopy, 62
        hyperopia, 47
        keratoscopy, 58–59
        kertaometry, 54–55
        pachymetry, 59–60
        retinoscopy, 46
        specular microscopy, 60
        trial frame refraction, 51–53
        ultrasonic scanning, 60–62

as LASIK complication, 131–132
    level of correction with refractive surgery, 31
Refractive surgery
    ametropia, limitations of, 175
    clear lens replacement, 153–159
    conjunctival abnormalities, 23–24
    contraindications for, 30–32, 69–70
    corneal disorders relevant to, 15–21
    extraocular muscles, 24–25
    eyelids, 22–23
    ignorance of, 31
    incisional techniques, 68–80
        astigmatic keratotomy (AK), 77–78
        limbal relaxing incisions (LRI), 79–80
        postoperative considerations, 72–73
        preoperative considerations, 68–69
        radial keratotomy (RK), 73–77
        surgical considerations, 69–72
    indications for, 28–30
    medical disorders relevant to, 10–15
    operative refractive targets, 64–67
    options for, 1–4
    orbital configuration and palpebral opening,
        25–26
    patient fear of, 30–31
    postoperative patient expectations, 32
    preoperative assessment, 28–35
    presbyopia, 214–217
    pupil size, 25
    retinal disorders, 26
    wavefront systems for, 147–152
Regression of effect, as radial keratotomy (RK)
        complication, 76
Regular astigmatism, classification and character-
        istics, 8
Reis Buckler corneal dystrophy, refractive surgery
        for patients with, 17
Retinal disorders, refractive surgery and, 26
Retinitis pigmentosa, fundus examination with, 44
Retinoscopy, postoperative refractive error assess-
        ment with, 46
Retreatment procedures, photorefractive keratec-
        tomy (PRK), 89–91
RK. *See* Radial keratotomy (RK)
Russian incision technique, radial keratotomy
        (RK), 74
Russian power calculations, phakic refractive lens
        implantation technique, 188

S
Scanning multipass technique, photorefractive
        keratectomy (PRK), 83–84
Schachar's theory, surgical reversal of presbyopia,
        215–216
Secondary ametropia, 6–7
Seidel's sums of optical aberrations of form, 144